Basic Pharmacokinetics Handbook

John R. White, Jr., Pharm.D.
Assistant Professor of Pharmacy Practice
College of Pharmacy
Washington State University
Spokane, Washington

Mark W. Garrison, Pharm.D.
Assistant Professor of Pharmacy Practice
College of Pharmacy
Washington State University
Spokane, Washington

Edited by
Mary Anne Koda-Kimble, Pharm.D.
Professor of Clinical Pharmacy
Chairwoman, Division of Clinical Pharmacy
School of Pharmacy
University of California
San Francisco, California

Applied Therapeutics, Inc.
Vancouver, WA

Applied Therapeutics, Inc.
Post Office Box 5077
Vancouver, Washington 98668-5077
(206) 253-7123

Library of Congress Catalog Card Number 94-71941
ISBN 0-915486-21-0

First Printing, December, 1994

This handbook is dedicated to Jane and Sue for their love, understanding, and support, and to our mentors at the University of California at San Francisco, Mercer University, and the University of Minnesota.

We would also like to extend our sincere appreciation to Nannette Naught, Linda Young, Michele Jobes, Rick Walsh, and the rest of the staff at Applied Therapeutics for their outstanding effort towards the creation of this first edition.

Notice to Reader

Drug therapy information is constantly evolving. Our ever-changing knowledge and experience with drugs and the continual development of new drugs necessitates changes in treatment and drug therapy. The editors, authors, and the publisher of this work have made every effort to ensure the information provided herein was accurate at the time of publication. *It remains the responsibility of every practitioner to evaluate the appropriateness of a particular opinion or therapy in the context of the actual clinical situation and with due consideration of any new developments in the field.* Although the author has been careful to recommend dosages that are in agreement with current standards and responsible literature, the student or practitioner should consult with several appropriate information sources when dealing with new and unfamiliar drugs.

Contents

Preface

This handbook is designed to serve as a practical guide and reference source for students and practitioners who understand the principles of pharmacokinetic theory, but who occasionally cannot recall the specific parameters and equations needed to perform pharmacokinetic evaluations of patients. The information presented is based on the approach and methods described by Michael E. Winter, Pharm.D. in his text, **Basic Clinical Pharmacokinetics**. Those who desire more background and explanation of clinical pharmacokinetics are referred to his text. Numbered equations presented in this handbook include cross references to corresponding equation and page numbers in Dr. Winter's text.

This handbook has two sections. Part I contains general information about pharmacokinetic equations, appropriate equation choice for a given situation, assessment of renal function, and the dialysis of drugs. Part II contains pharmacokinetic monographs for individual drugs. Although pharmacokinetic equations can be used to calculate the dose of a particular drug, it is imperative that the practitioner take a common sense approach to the clinical application of pharmacokinetic principles. Before making dosage recommendations, the clinician must determine whether the calculated dose seems reasonable and rational within the specific context of the patient in question.

Equations

The following equations are arranged to solve for plasma drug concentration (Cp). This arrangement is used for consistency only. The pharmacokineticist frequently uses known concentration data to solve for patient-specific parameters in the clinical setting. For information on manipulation of these equations and revision of patient parameters see **Basic Clinical Pharmacokinetics**, 3rd edition.

First-Order Equations

$$Kd = \frac{\ln\left(\dfrac{Cp_1}{Cp_2}\right)}{t}$$

(Eq. 1)
(Eq 28, pg 41)

$$Kd = \frac{Cl}{Vd}$$

(Eq. 2)
(Eq 27, pg 41)

$$Kd = \frac{0.693}{t\frac{1}{2}}$$

(Eq. 3)
(Eq 8.4, pg 277)

Elimination Rate Constant (Kd). The elimination rate constant (Kd) relates to the fractional rate of drug loss from the body. It may also be viewed as the fraction of the volume of distribution that is cleared of drug during a time interval. The Kd for a drug which exhibits first-order elimination is equal to the slope of the line produced when the ln concentration is plotted versus time. (See Equation 1 and Figure 1.) First-order elimination data plotted on a non-logarithmic graph is curvilinear. (See Figure 2.) The Kd in Figure 1 can be calculated from any two time points. For example, using Equation 1:

$$Kd = \frac{\ln\left(\dfrac{70.7}{50.0}\right)}{1 \text{ hr}}$$

$$= 0.347 \text{ hr}^{-1}$$

Half-Life (t½)

$$t\frac{1}{2} = \frac{0.693}{Kd}$$

(Eq. 4)
(Eq 31, pg 43)

$$t\frac{1}{2} = \frac{(0.693)(Vd)}{Cl}$$

(Eq. 5)
(Eq 32, pg 43)

Half-life (t½) is the time required for the concentration of a drug that is eliminated by a first-order process to be reduced by one half. The t½ in Figure 1 can be directly determined by evaluation

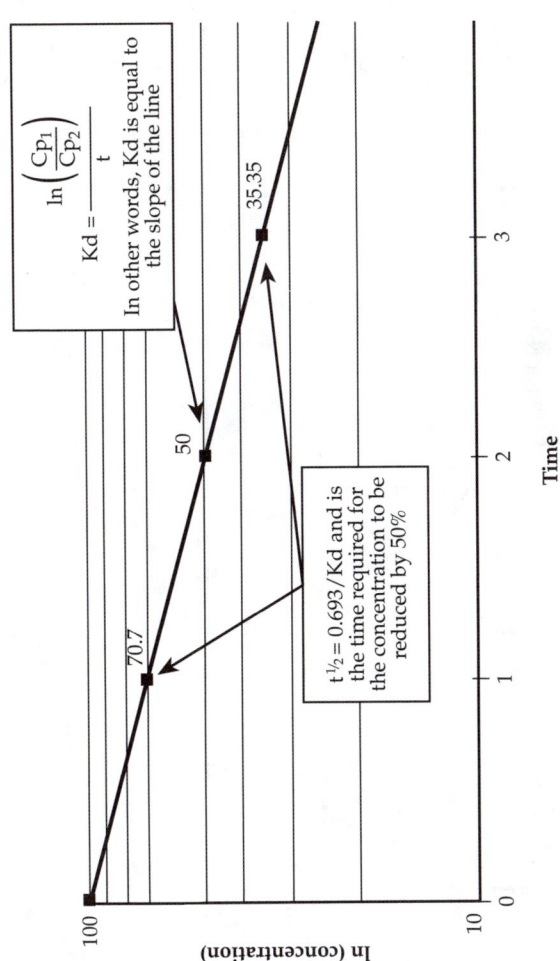

Figure 1. First order elimination: ln concentration versus time.

$$Kd = \frac{\ln\left(\frac{Cp_1}{Cp_2}\right)}{t}$$

In other words, Kd is equal to the slope of the line

$t\frac{1}{2} = 0.693 / Kd$ and is the time required for the concentration to be reduced by 50%

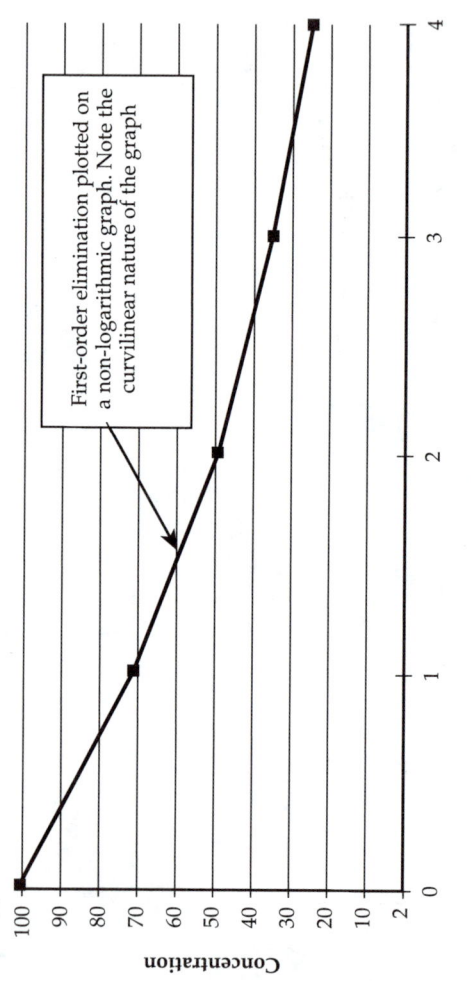

The box within the figure reads:

First-order elimination plotted on a non-logarithmic graph. Note the curvilinear nature of the graph

Figure 2. First order elimination: concentration versus time.

of the straight line plotted, or it can be calculated by the use of an equation. For example, using Equation 4:

$$t^{1/2} = \frac{0.693}{0.347 \ hr^{-1}}$$

$$= 2 \ hr$$

Volume of Distribution (Vd)

$$Vd = \frac{Dose}{Cp_{initial}} \qquad \textbf{(Eq. 6)}$$

$$Vd = \frac{Cl}{Kd} \qquad \textbf{(Eq. 7)}$$

The apparent volume of distribution can be calculated by dividing the dose by the initial concentration after an IV bolus (Equation 6), or it can be calculated based on the relationship cited in Equation 7 when Cl and Kd are known. In Figure 3, a 1500 mg IV bolus produced an initial concentration of 100 mg/L. The calculated volume is 1500 mg/(100 mg/L) or 15 L.

Single IV Bolus Dose

$$Cp_1 = \frac{(S)(F)(Loading \ Dose)}{Vd} \ (e^{-Kdt_1}) \qquad \textbf{(Eq. 8)}$$

(Eq 50, pg 57)

where: $\dfrac{(S)(F)(\text{Loading Dose})}{Vd}$ = Initial concentration

$\quad\quad (e^{-Kdt_1})$ = Fraction remaining at t_1 after the dose

This equation can be used to determine a concentration at any time after a single IV bolus dose has been administered. For example, given the following data concerning Figure 3, the concentration 4 hr after the dose could be calculated by using Equation 8.

Given that:
Dose = 1500 mg
F = 1
S = 1
Vd = 15 L
Kd = 0.346 hr^{-1}

Concentration 4 hr after dose

$$Cp_1 = \frac{(1)(1)(1500 \text{ mg})}{15 \text{ L}}\,(e^{-(0.346)(4)})$$

$$= 25 \text{ mg/L}$$

Nonsteady-State Intermittent IV Bolus

$$Cp_2 = \frac{\dfrac{(S)(F)(\text{Dose})}{Vd}}{(1 - e^{-Kd\tau})}\,(1 - e^{-Kd(N)\tau})(e^{-Kdt_2})$$

(Eq. 9)

(Eq 55, pg 68)

where: $\dfrac{(S)(F)(Dose)}{Vd}$ = Concentration change elicited by each dose

$(1 - e^{-Kd\tau})$ = Fraction of drug lost in the dosing interval. When used in the denominator, this fraction compensates for drug that accumulates during the interval; the "accumulation factor"

$\dfrac{\dfrac{(S)(F)(Dose)}{Vd}}{1 - e^{-Kd\tau}}$ = Cpss max or peak concentration at steady state

$(1 - e^{-Kd(N)\tau})$ = Describes the fraction of steady state achieved after N doses have been administered

(e^{-Kdt_2}) = Fraction remaining at t_2 or the number of hours since the last dose

This equation is useful in situations where multiple intermittent IV bolus doses have been administered, but steady-state peaks and troughs have not been achieved (i.e., <3–5 $t\frac{1}{2}$s have elapsed). Use of this equation assumes that the dose, the dosing interval, and patient clinical parameters have remained unchanged during the period of time in question. It is most appropriate to use this equation to predict concentrations produced by the first 3 or 4 doses in Figure 4. Peaks and troughs have reached a steady-state plateau after the fifth dose. This equation can also be used in a nonsteady-state, intermittent short infusion situation when the amount of drug lost during the infusion is negligible (i.e., t_{in} <⅛ $t\frac{1}{2}$). For

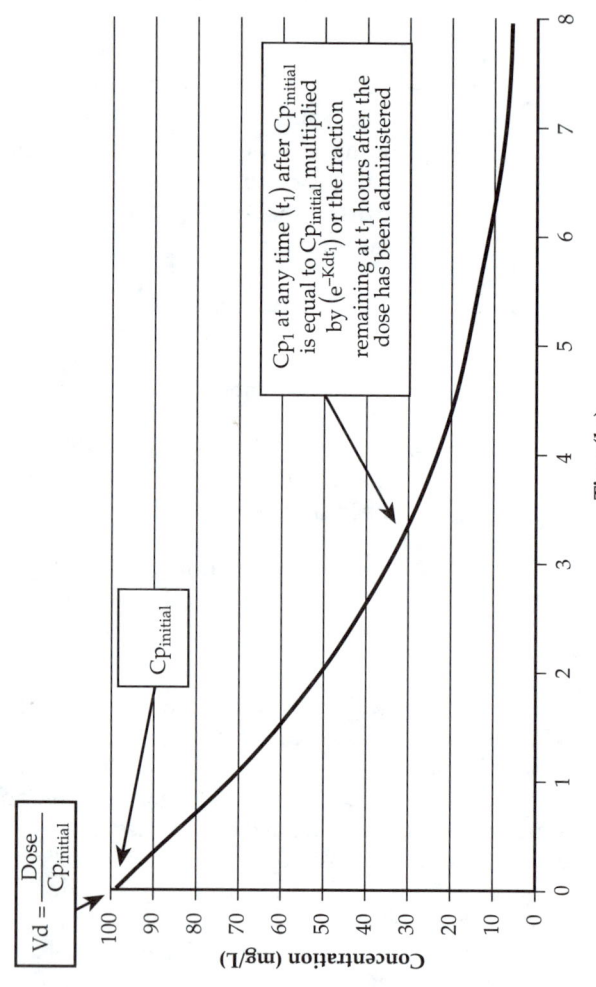

Figure 3. Single IV bolus dose. D = 1500 mg, Vd = 15 L, Kd = 0.346 hr^{-1}.

$Vd = \dfrac{Dose}{Cp_{initial}}$

$Cp_{initial}$

Cp_1 at any time (t_1) after $Cp_{initial}$ is equal to $Cp_{initial}$ multiplied by (e^{-Kdt_1}) or the fraction remaining at t_1 hours after the dose has been administered

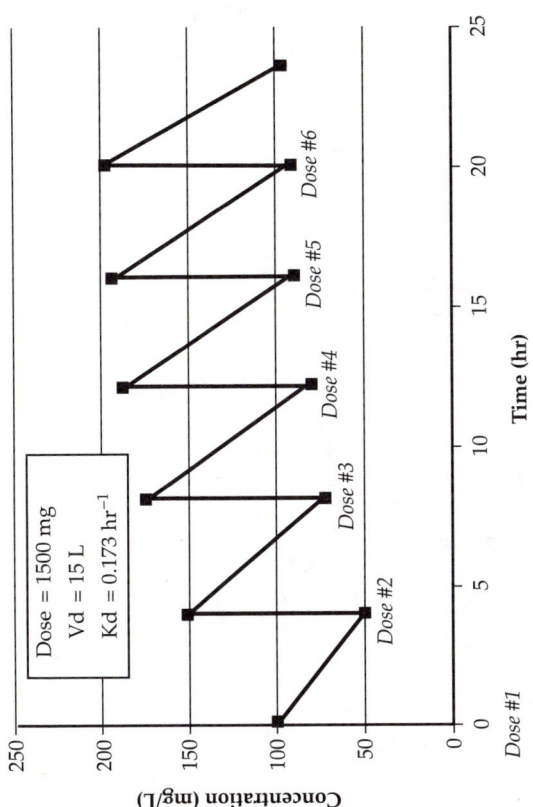

Figure 4. Intermittent IV bolus doses. D = 150 mg, Vd = 15 L, Kd = 0.173 hr^{-1}.

example, given the data below in the situation depicted in Figure 4, the peak and the trough (4 hr after the dose) concentrations can be predicted after the second dose.

$$
\begin{aligned}
\text{Given that:} \quad (S)(F)(Dose) &= 1500 \text{ mg} \\
Vd &= 15 \text{ L} \\
Kd &= 0.173 \text{ hr}^{-1} \\
N &= 2 \\
\tau &= 4 \text{ hr}
\end{aligned}
$$

Peak concentration

$$
\begin{aligned}
Cp &= \frac{\dfrac{1500 \text{ mg}}{15 \text{ L}}}{(1 - e^{-(0.173)(4)})} \left(1 - e^{-(0.173)(2)(4)}\right)\left(e^{-(0.173)(0)}\right) \\
&= \frac{100 \text{ mg/L}}{(0.5)} (0.75)\,(1) \\
&= 150 \text{ mg/L}
\end{aligned}
$$

Trough concentration

$$
\begin{aligned}
Cp &= 150 \text{ mg/L} \left(e^{-(0.173)(4)}\right) \\
&= 75 \text{ mg/L}
\end{aligned}
$$

Steady-State Intermittent IV Bolus

$$
Cpss_1 = \frac{\dfrac{(S)(F)(Dose)}{Vd}}{(1 - e^{-Kd\tau})} \left(e^{-Kdt_1}\right)
$$

(Eq. 10)

(Eq 48, pg 56)

where: $\dfrac{(S)(F)(Dose)}{Vd}$ = Concentration of change elicited by each dose

$(1 - e^{-Kd\tau})$ = When used in the denominator, this fraction compensates for drug that accumulates during the interval

(e^{-Kdt_1}) = Fraction remaining at t_1 time after the dose

This equation is appropriate in situations when intermittent IV bolus doses have been administered at a constant interval for 3–5 $t\frac{1}{2}$s. (*Note:* The dose must be constant.) This equation may also be used in a steady-state intermittent short infusion situation when the amount of drug lost during the infusion is negligible (i.e., t_{in} <$\frac{1}{8}$ $t\frac{1}{2}$). For example, given the following data concerning the situation in Figure 4, the peak and trough concentrations can be predicted.

Given that: $(S)(F)(Dose) = 1500$ mg
$Vd = 15$ L
$Kd = 0.173$ hr^{-1}
$t = 4$ hr

Peak concentration

$$Cp = \dfrac{\dfrac{1500 \text{ mg}}{15 \text{ L}}}{(1 - e^{-(0.173)(4)})}$$

$$= 200 \text{ mg/L}$$

Trough concentration

$$Cp = 200 \text{ mg/L } (e^{-(0.173)(4)})$$

$$= 100 \text{ mg/L}$$

Nonsteady-State Continuous Infusion

$$Cp_1 = \frac{(S)(F)(Dose/\tau)}{Cl} (1 - e^{-Kdt_{in}}) \qquad \textbf{(Eq. 11)}$$

(Eq 37, pg 48)

where: $\dfrac{(S)(F)(Dose/\tau)}{Cl}$ = Average steady-state concentration

$(1 - e^{-Kdt_{in}})$ = Fraction of steady state achieved any time t_1 after starting the infusion

This equation is used in situations when a continuous infusion is being administered, but the concentration has not reached steady state (i.e., <3–5 t½s have elapsed). In Figure 5 this equation is appropriate to use before the 16–20 hr time point.

The example in Figure 5 depicts a drug which is administered at a rate of 500 mg/hr, has a Cl = 5.0 L/hr, and an elimination rate constant of 0.231 hr^{-1}. The concentration at 5 hr (t_{in}) can be predicted using Equation 11.

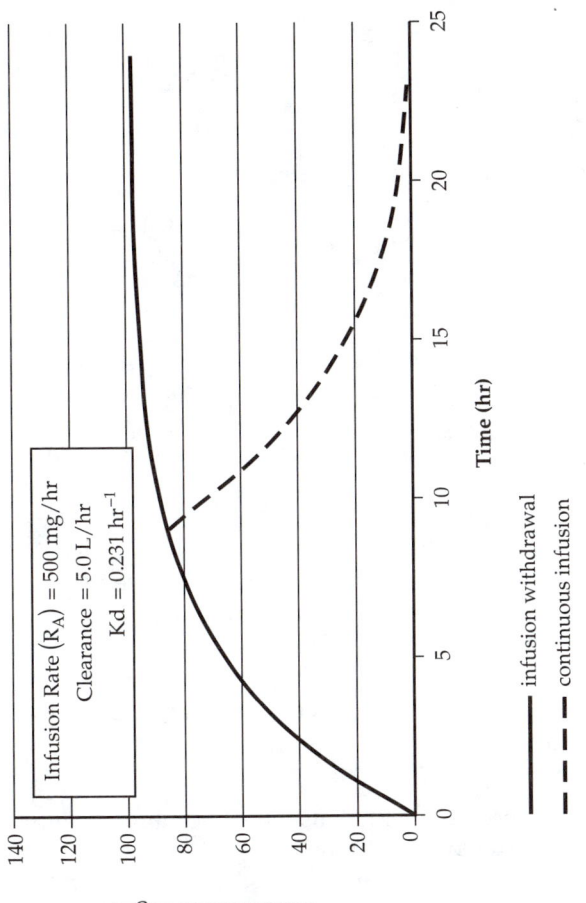

Figure 5. Continuous infusion. $D/\tau = 500$ mg/hr, $Cl = 5$ L/hr, $Kd = 0.231$ hr^{-1}.

Infusion Rate $(R_A) = 500$ mg/hr

Clearance $= 5.0$ L/hr

$Kd = 0.231$ hr^{-1}

Time (hr)

Concentration (mg/L)

—— infusion withdrawal

- - - continuous infusion

$$Cp_1 = \frac{500 \text{ mg/hr}}{5.0 \text{ L/hr}} (1 - e^{-(0.231)(5)})$$

$$= (100 \text{ mg/L})(0.68)$$

$$= 68 \text{ mg/L}$$

Decay After Nonsteady-State Continuous Infusion

$$Cp_2 = \frac{(S)(F)(\text{Dose}/\tau)}{Cl} (1 - e^{-Kdt_{in}})(e^{-Kdt_2})$$ **(Eq. 12)**

(Eq 41, pg 49)

where: $\dfrac{(S)(F)(\text{Dose}/\tau)}{Cl}$ = Average steady-state concentration

$(1 - e^{-Kdt_{in}})$ = Describes the fraction of steady state achieved t_1 hr after starting the infusion

(e^{-Kdt_2}) = Fraction remaining at t_2 hr after the end of the infusion

This equation is useful in situations when a continuous infusion has been administered and the infusion is discontinued before steady-state conditions have been reached. (See Figure 5.) For example, if the infusion was discontinued after 9 hr (t_1), the concentration 6 hr later (t_2) could be predicted as follows:

$$Cp_2 = \frac{500 \text{ mg/hr}}{5.0 \text{ L/hr}} (1 - e^{-(0.231)(9)})(e^{-(0.231)(6)})$$

$$= 100 \text{ mg/L}(0.87)(0.25)$$

$$= 21.75 \text{ mg/L}$$

Steady-State Continuous Infusion

$$Cpss \text{ ave} = \frac{(S)(F)(Dose/\tau)}{Cl} = \frac{R_A}{Cl} \qquad \textbf{(Eq. 13)}$$
$$\text{(Eq 35, pg 46)}$$

This equation is appropriate in situations when a continuous infusion is continued until a steady-state concentration has been achieved. This equation can also be useful in situations of intermittent drug administration when the interval is $<\frac{1}{2}$ t½. In this situation, Cpss min, Cpss ave, and Cpss max may not be significantly different. For example, in Figure 5, when the dose is 500 mg/hr and the Cl is 5 L/hr, the predicted Cpss ave is 100 mg/L.

$$Cpss \text{ ave} = \frac{500 \text{ mg/hr}}{5.0 \text{ L/hr}}$$

$$= 100 \text{ mg/L}$$

The concentration at any time after the end of the infusion (i.e., after steady state is reached) can be predicted by multiplying the Cpss ave by (e^{-Kdt_1}).

Single Short Infusion

$$Cp_2 = \frac{(S)(F)(Dose/t_{in})}{Cl} (1 - e^{-Kdt_{in}})(e^{-Kdt_2}) \quad \textbf{(Eq. 14)}$$

(Eq 53, pg 63)

where: $\dfrac{(S)(F)(Dose/t_{in})}{Cl}$ = Average steady-state concentration that would be achieved if the drug were administered continuously

$(1 - e^{-Kdt_{in}})$ = Fraction of the above mentioned steady-state average concentration that is achieved after the short infusion

(e^{-Kdt_2}) = Fraction remaining at t_2 time after the end of the infusion

This equation is appropriate when a single dose of medication has been administered by short infusion and the amount of drug lost during the infusion is significant. The peak and trough concentration after the first dose (see Figure 6) can be calculated given the following information.

Given that: $(S)(F)(Dose) = 1000$ mg

$t_{in} = 1$ hr

$Kd = 0.231$ hr^{-1}

$Cl = 2.05$ L/hr

Peak concentration

$$Cp = \frac{1000 \text{ mg/hr}}{2.05 \text{ L/hr}} (1 - e^{-(0.231)(1)})$$

$$= 487 \text{ mg/L } (0.2)$$

$$= 98 \text{ mg/L}$$

Trough concentration

$$Cp = 98 \text{ mg/L } (e^{-(0.231)(3)})$$

$$= 49 \text{ mg/L}$$

Note: The number used here is 3 hr, not 4 hr. Although sampling occurs 4 hr from the beginning of the infusion, this equation predicts the concentration x hr after the infusion has *ended*.

Nonsteady-State Intermittent Short Infusion

$$Cp = \frac{\dfrac{(S)(F)(Dose/t_{in})}{Cl} (1 - e^{-Kdt_{in}})}{(1 - e^{-Kd\tau})} (1 - e^{-Kd(N)\tau})(e^{-Kdt_2})$$

(Eq. 15)
(Eq 56, pg 68)

where: $\dfrac{(S)(F)(Dose/t_{in})}{Cl}$ = Steady-state average concentration that would be achieved if the drug were administered continuously

$(1 - e^{-Kdt_{in}})$ = Fraction of the above mentioned steady-state average concentration that is achieved after one short infusion

$(1 - e^{-Kd\tau})$ = Fraction of the drug lost during the interval. When used as a denominator, this fraction takes into account the accumulation of drug between doses

$(1 - e^{-Kd(N)\tau})$ = Fraction of steady state achieved after N doses have been administered at a fixed interval

$(1 - e^{-Kdt_2})$ = Fraction remaining at time t_2 after the end of the infusion

This equation is useful in situations when multiple short infusions of a drug have been administered at a constant dose and interval before achieving steady-state conditions. For example, the peak and trough concentrations after the second dose in Figure 6 can be calculated as follows:

Peak concentration

$$Cp = \frac{\dfrac{1000 \text{ mg}/1 \text{ hr}}{2.05 \text{ L/hr}}}{(1 - e^{-(0.231)(4)})} (1 - e^{-(0.231)(2)(4)})(1 - e^{-(0.231)(1)})$$

$$= \frac{488 \text{ mg/L}}{0.6} (0.84)(0.2)$$

$$= 137 \text{ mg/L}$$

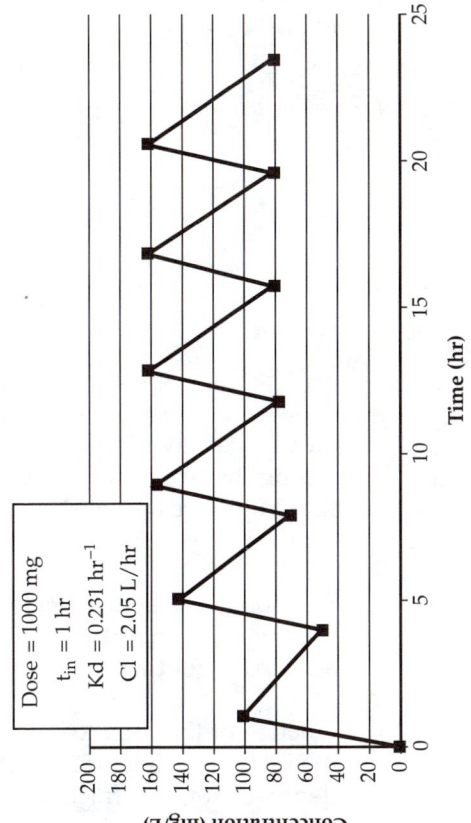

Figure 6. Intermittent short infusion. $D/t_{in} = 1000$ mg/hr, $t_{in} = 1$ hr, $Kd = 0.231$ hr^{-1}, $Cl = 2.05$ L/hr.

Dose = 1000 mg
$t_{in} = 1$ hr
$Kd = 0.231$ hr^{-1}
$Cl = 2.05$ L/hr

Trough concentration

$$Cp = 137 \text{ mg/L} \left(e^{-(0.231)(3)}\right)$$

$$= 69 \text{ mg/L}$$

Steady-State Intermittent Short Infusion

$$Cpss_2 = \frac{\dfrac{(S)(F)(Dose/t_{in})}{Cl}\left(1 - e^{-Kdt_{in}}\right)}{\left(1 - e^{-Kd\tau}\right)}\left(e^{-Kdt_2}\right)$$

(Eq. 16)
(Eq 57, pg 69)

where: $\dfrac{(S)(F)(Dose/t_{in})}{Cl}$ = Steady-state average concentration that would be achieved if the drug were administered continuously

$(1 - e^{-Kdt_{in}})$ = Fraction of the above mentioned steady-state concentration achieved after the short infusion

$(1 - e^{-Kd\tau})$ = Fraction of the drug lost during the interval. When used as the denominator, this fraction takes into consideration the accumulation of drug between doses

(e^{-Kdt_2}) = Fraction remaining at time t_2 after the end of the infusion

This equation is useful in situations when multiple short infusions of a drug have been administered at a constant dose and interval for more than 3–5 t½s. For example, the peak and trough concentrations after steady state has been achieved in Figure 6 can be calculated as follows:

Peak concentration

$$Cp = \frac{\dfrac{1000 \text{ mg}/1 \text{ hr}}{2.05 \text{ L/hr}}}{(1 - e^{-(0.231)(4)})} (1 - e^{-(0.231)(1)})$$

$$= \frac{488 \text{ mg/L}}{0.6} (0.2)$$

$$= 163 \text{ mg/L}$$

Trough concentration

$$Cp = 163 \text{ mg/L} (e^{-(0.231)(3)})$$

$$= 82 \text{ mg/L}$$

Nonlinear Equations

Dose to Produce a Target Average Steady-State Concentration

$$(S)(F)(Dose/\tau) = \frac{(Vm)(Cpss \text{ ave})}{Km + Cpss \text{ ave}} \quad \textbf{(Eq. 17)}$$

(Eq 10.5, pg 318)

When using this equation one must either: 1) assume average values for Vm and Km from the literature or 2) use patient-specific parameters calculated from previous steady-state concentrations. Given the following phenytoin parameters and patient characteristics, the dose required to produce a Cpss ave of 10 mg/L may be calculated.

Given that: Patient weight = 55 kg

$$Vm = 7 \text{ mg/kg/day or } 385 \text{ mg/day}$$

$$S = 0.92 \text{ (assuming the use of phenytoin capsules)}$$

$$F = 1.0$$

Dose Required to Produce Cpss ave of 10 mg/L

$$(S)(F)(Dose/\tau) = \frac{(385 \text{ mg/day})(10 \text{ mg/L})}{(4 \text{ mg/L} + 10 \text{ mg/L})}$$

$$(S)(F)(Dose/\tau) = 275 \text{ mg/day}$$

$$\frac{\text{Best Dose Based Upon}}{\text{Available Dosage Forms}} = 299 \text{ mg/day or } 300 \text{ mg/day}$$

Prediction of Steady-State Plasma Concentration

$$\text{Cpss ave} = \frac{(Km)[(S)(F)(Dose/\tau)]}{Vm - (S)(F)(Dose/\tau)} \quad \textbf{(Eq. 18)}$$

(Eq 10.6, pg 318)

When using this equation one must either: 1) assume that the patient's values for Vm and Km are similar to average values from the literature or 2) use patient-specific parameters calculated from previous steady-state concentrations. Using the above parameters, the Cpss ave in the patient taking 300 mg/day of phenytoin capsules can be predicted as follows:

$$\text{Cpss ave} = \frac{(4 \text{ mg/L})[(0.92)(300/1)]}{385 - (0.92)(300/1)}$$

$$= 10 \text{ mg/L}$$

Mass Balance Equations

$$\frac{\text{Amount Eliminated}}{t} = (S)(F)(\text{Dose}/\tau) - \left[\frac{(Cp_2 - Cp_1)(Vd)}{t}\right]$$

(Eq. 19)

(Eq 10.21, pg 333)

$$Vm = \frac{\left[\dfrac{\text{Amount Eliminated}}{t}\right]\left[Km + \left(\dfrac{Cp_1 + Cp_2}{2}\right)\right]}{\left(\dfrac{Cp_1 + Cp_2}{2}\right)}$$

(Eq. 20)

(Eq. 10.22, pg 334)

The above equations can be used to predict patient-specific parameters in the absence of steady-state concentration data. To use the above equations, one must have the following data:

⇨ 1. Two plasma concentrations.

⇨ 2. The time change between the two concentrations (t).

⇨ 3. The amount of drug administered during the interval.

The amount eliminated over the interval is calculated in Equation 19 and inserted into Equation 20 to yield a specific Vm; Km must be assumed. For example, given the following nonsteady-state data, one could proceed as follows.

$$\text{Patient weight} = 60 \text{ kg}$$

$$Vd = 0.65 \text{ L/kg or } 39 \text{ L}$$
for this patient

$$\text{Dose} = \text{Patient has been receiving}$$
360 mg/day of sodium phenytoin
for the past 5 days

$$Cp_1 = 10 \text{ mg/L}$$
(at the beginning of the 5-day period)

$$Cp_2 = 15 \text{ mg/L}$$
(at the end of the 5-day period)

Note: Cp_1 and Cp_2 are nonsteady-state concentrations.

$$\frac{\text{Amount Eliminated}}{t} = (0.92)(360/1 \text{ day}) - \frac{(15 - 10)(39)}{5 \text{ days}}$$

$$= 331 \text{ mg} - 39 \text{ mg}$$

$$= 292 \text{ mg/day}$$

$$Vm = \frac{\left[292 \text{ mg/day}\right]\left(4 + \dfrac{10 + 15}{2}\right)}{\left(\dfrac{10 + 15}{2}\right)}$$

$$= 385 \text{ mg/day}$$

This patient-specific Vm of 385 mg/day could then be used in Equation 17 to predict a new maintenance dose to yield a desired Cpss ave. For example, the daily dose needed to maintain this patient at a Cpss ave of 15 mg/L can be calculated as follows:

$$(0.92)(F)(Dose/\tau) = \frac{(385 \text{ mg/day})(15 \text{ mg/L})}{4 \text{ mg/L} + 15 \text{ mg/L}}$$

$$= 330 \text{ mg/day}$$

Adjustment for Plasma Protein Binding

$$Cp_{\text{Normal Binding}} = \frac{Cp'}{(1 - \alpha)\left[\dfrac{P'}{P_{NL}}\right] + \alpha}$$

(Eq. 21)
(Eq 8, pg 12)

where: α = Free fraction

        Cp' = Plasma concentration measured in patients with decreased plasma protein binding

        P' = Patient's serum albumin concentration in mg/dL

        P_{NL} = 4.4 mg/dL average normal serum albumin

This equation normalizes phenytoin concentrations in patients with abnormally low serum albumin concentrations. It yields an estimate of the patient's expected phenytoin concentration if that patient's serum albumin levels were normal. This normalization accounts for the increase in free concentration of drug (active form) that accompanies a decrease in available binding sites. For example, if a patient with a serum phenytoin concentration of 7 mg/L had a serum albumin level of 1.9 mg/dL, the phenytoin value would be normalized as follows:

$$Cp_{\text{Normal Binding}} = \frac{7 \text{ mg/L}}{(1 - 0.1)\left[\dfrac{1.9}{4.4}\right] + 0.1}$$

$$= 14.28 \text{ mg/L}$$

Note: α for phenytoin $= 0.1$; $P_{NL} = 4.4$ mg/dL.

This suggests that this patient's phenytoin concentration of 7 mg/L has the therapeutic effectiveness of a concentration of 14.2 mg/L in a patient with normal binding. An adjustment in dose would probably not be warranted in this case.

Adjustment for Plasma Protein
Binding in a Patient with $Cl_{Cr} <10$ mL/min

$$Cp_{\text{Normal Binding}} = \frac{Cp'}{(0.48)(1 - \alpha)\left(\dfrac{P'}{P_{NL}}\right) + \alpha}$$

(Eq. 22)
(Eq 10.2, pg 315)

The affinity of phenytoin for albumin is decreased in the presence of severe renal failure. This equation adjusts phenytoin concentrations in patients with abnormally low serum albumin concentrations and co-existing renal failure (Cl_{Cr} = <10 mL/min). The binding of phenytoin to plasma protein binding sites is decreased by some factor (not yet elucidated) which accompanies renal failure. Protein binding may be altered in patients with Cl_{Cr} values ranging from 10–25 mL/min, but is not altered in a predictable manner. Lastly, this equation may be used in those with normal albumin concentrations who have Cl_{Cr} <10 mL/min.

Notes:

Notes:

Choice of Equations

The following flow chart can be used to determine the appropriate equation for a given situation. Although the selection of an equation may at first seem obvious based on its name, closer inspection of clinical situations reveals that the choice may not be based on equation name alone. For example, the continuous infusion equation can be used to predict the concentration of phenobarbital in a patient who takes phenobarbital orally QD. In this situation, the half-life (t½) of phenobarbital is long relative to its dosing interval, and significant peak to trough variance would not be expected. Similarly, the intermittent IV bolus model can be a reasonable equation to use in a situation when the medication is administered by intermittent short infusion, but the t½ is relatively long since little drug is lost during the infusion. To determine the appropriate equation model for a given situation, simply answer the questions in the flow chart and continue until an equation is reached at the endpoint.

Algorithm for Choosing the Appropriate Pharmacokinetic Model

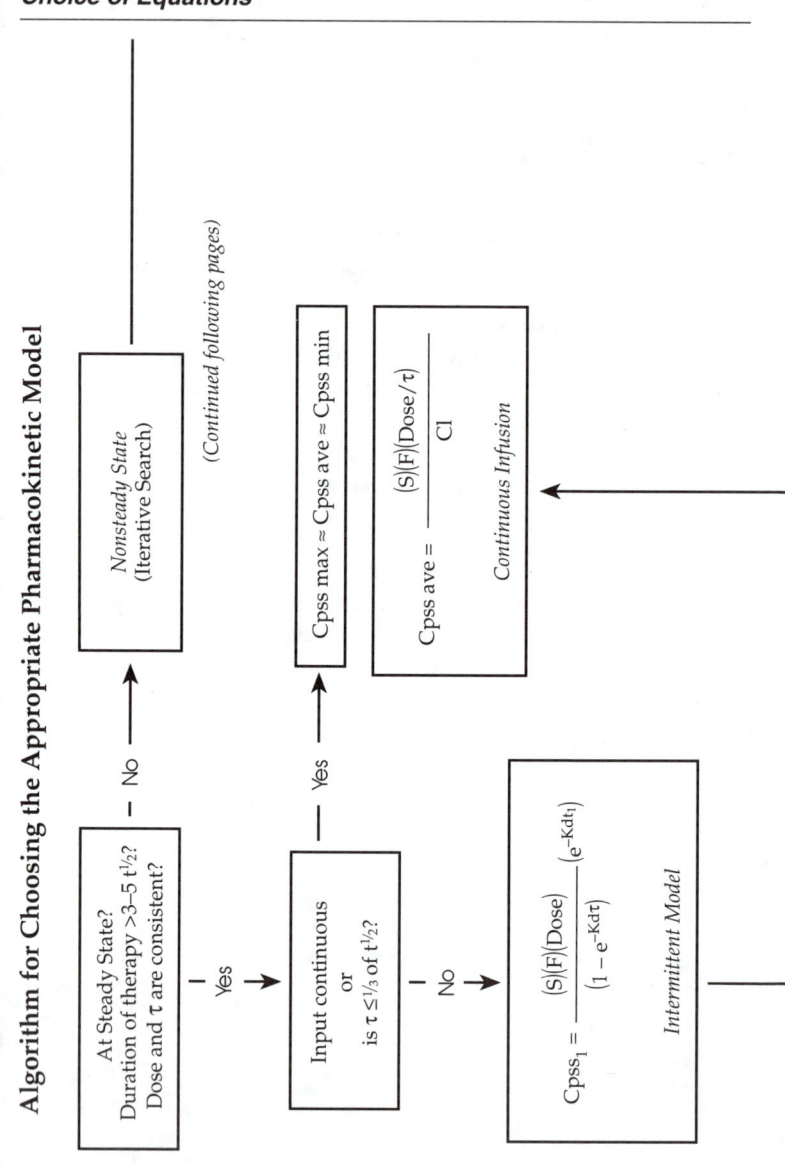

At Steady State?
Duration of therapy >3–5 t½?
Dose and τ are consistent?

— No → *Nonsteady State*
(Iterative Search)

(Continued following pages)

Yes ↓

Input continuous
or
is τ ≤⅓ of t½?

— Yes → Cpss max ≈ Cpss ave ≈ Cpss min

$$\text{Cpss ave} = \frac{(S)(F)(\text{Dose}/\tau)}{Cl}$$

Continuous Infusion

— No →

$$\text{Cpss}_1 = \frac{(S)(F)(\text{Dose})}{(1 - e^{-Kd\tau})} (e^{-Kdt_1})$$

Intermittent Model

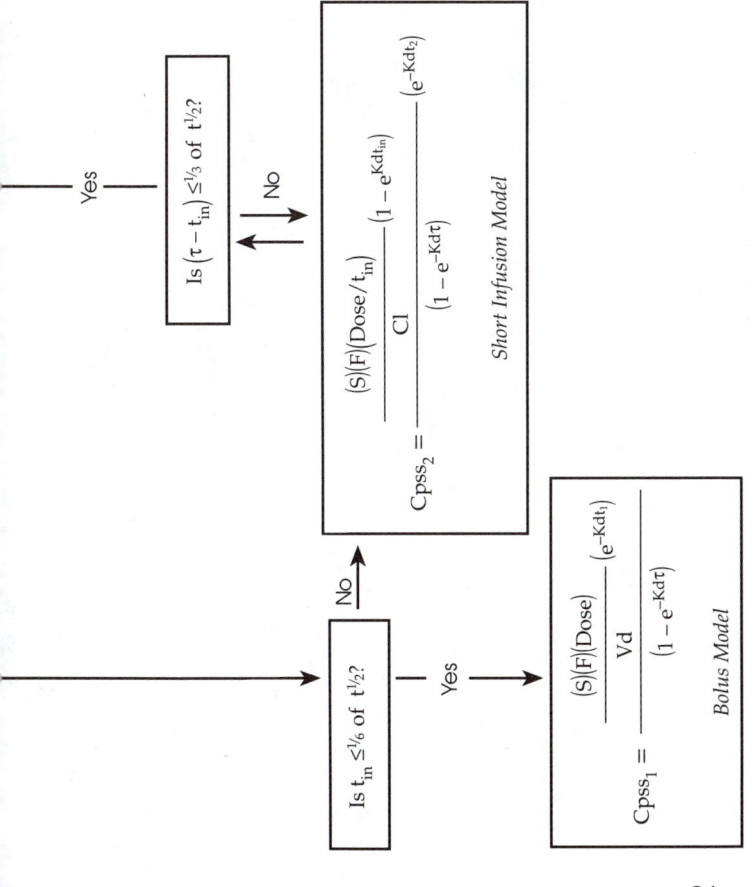

Algorithm for Choosing the Appropriate Pharmacokinetic Model
(Continued)

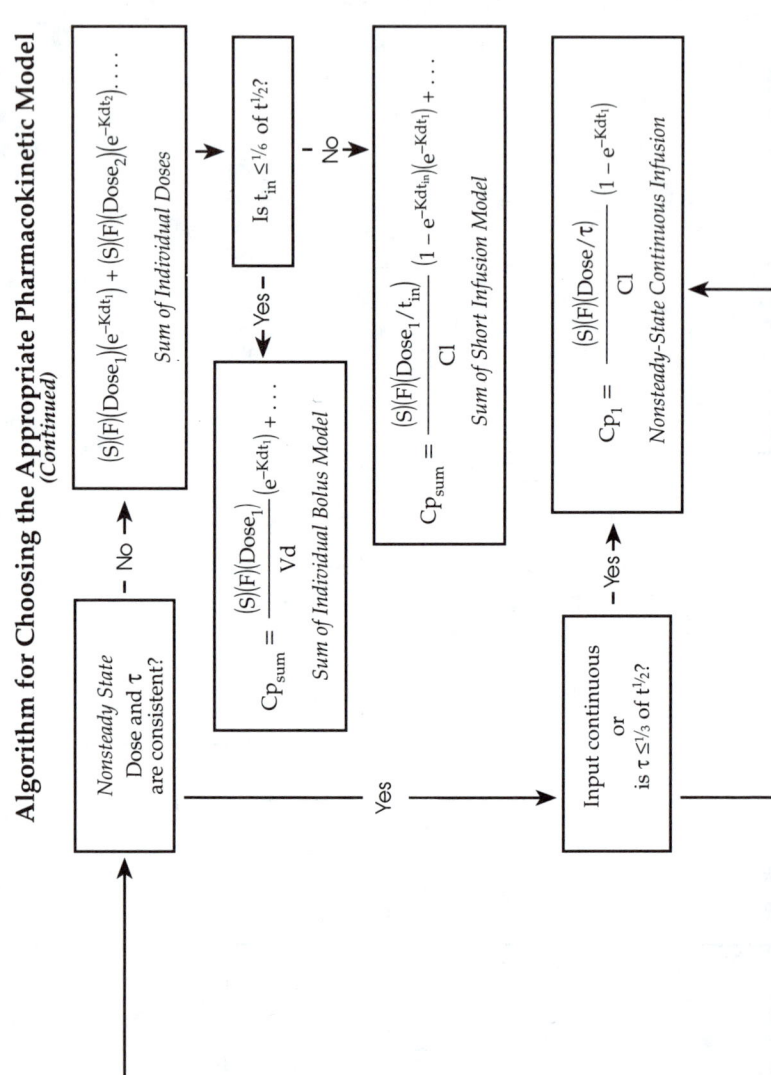

Nonsteady State
Dose and τ
are consistent?

— No →

$(S)(F)(Dose_1)(e^{-Kdt_1}) + (S)(F)(Dose_2)(e^{-Kdt_2})\cdots$

Sum of Individual Doses

Is $t_{in} \leq \frac{1}{6}$ of $t^{1/2}$?

→ No →

— Yes —

$$Cp_{sum} = \frac{(S)(F)(Dose_1)}{Vd}(e^{-Kdt_1}) + \cdots$$

Sum of Individual Bolus Model

$$Cp_{sum} = \frac{(S)(F)(Dose_1/t_{in})}{Cl}(1 - e^{-Kdt_{in}})(e^{-Kdt_1}) + \cdots$$

Sum of Short Infusion Model

$$Cp_1 = \frac{(S)(F)(Dose/\tau)}{Cl}(1 - e^{-Kdt_1})$$

Nonsteady-State Continuous Infusion

Yes

Input continuous
or is $\tau \leq \frac{1}{3}$ of $t^{1/2}$?

— Yes →

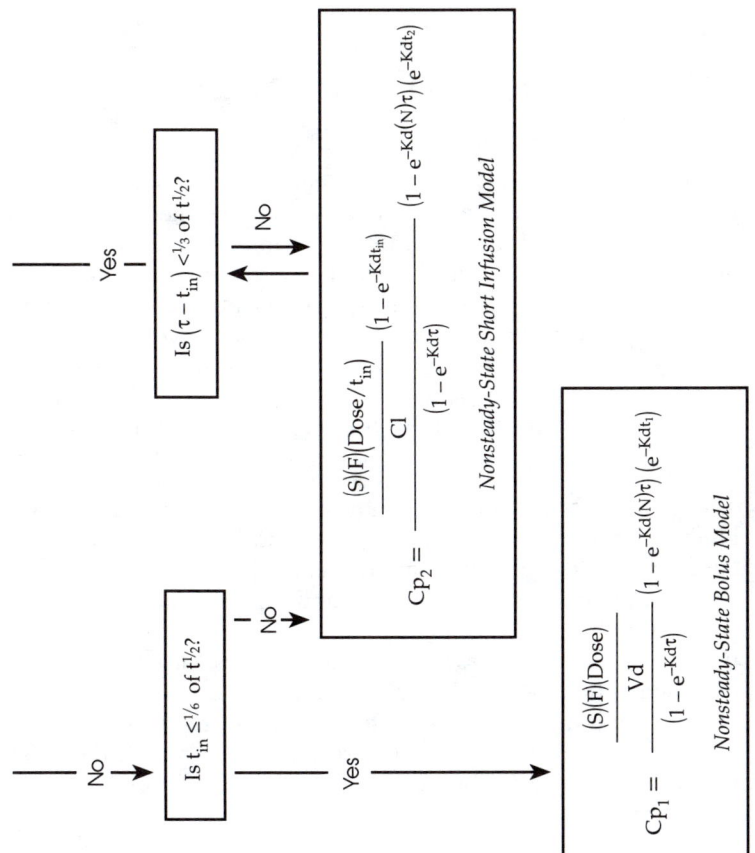

Is $\left(\tau - t_{in}\right) < \frac{1}{3}$ of $t^{1/2}$?

Yes

No

$$Cp_2 = \dfrac{\dfrac{(S)(F)(Dose/t_{in})}{Cl}\ (1 - e^{-Kdt_{in}})}{(1 - e^{-Kd\tau})}\ (1 - e^{-Kd(N)\tau})\ (e^{-Kdt_2})$$

Nonsteady-State Short Infusion Model

Is $t_{in} \leq \frac{1}{6}$ of $t^{1/2}$?

No

No →

Yes

$$Cp_1 = \dfrac{\dfrac{(S)(F)(Dose)}{Vd}}{(1 - e^{-Kd\tau})}\ (1 - e^{-Kd(N)\tau})\ (e^{-Kdt_1})$$

Nonsteady-State Bolus Model

Assessment of Renal Function

The clinical pharmacokineticist often must estimate renal function because many medications are cleared by renal mechanisms. An assessment of renal function can also be important for drugs that are cleared entirely by hepatic mechanisms because their disposition can also be altered by changes in renal function. For example, phenytoin is metabolized hepatically; however, its protein binding, volume of distribution (Vd), and plasma concentration (Cp) are all altered in patients with renal failure. Evaluation of renal function in the acutely ill patient is significant in almost all cases.

The renal clearance of drugs can be divided into three processes: glomerular filtration, tubular secretion, and tubular reabsorption. Glomerular filtration occurs at an average rate of 120 mL/min in a 70 kg individual. Drugs that are bound to plasma proteins cannot pass through the glomerular filtrate because the normal glomerulus does not allow passage of macromolecules. Tubular secretion is an active process which affects both bound and unbound molecules. The clearance of medication by the secretory pathway is offset to varying degrees by reabsorption. The net clearance of medications via the kidneys is described by the following equation:

$$\frac{\text{Rate of}}{\text{Excretion}} = \frac{\text{Rate of}}{\text{Filtration}} + \frac{\text{Rate of}}{\text{Secretion}} - \frac{\text{Rate of}}{\text{Absorption}} \qquad \textbf{(Eq. 23)}[2]$$

In the clinical setting, it is very difficult to assess tubular secretory rates or the amount of drug reabsorbed; however, creatinine clearance (Cl_{Cr}) closely approximates the glomerular filtration rate and can be estimated by a number of relatively pragmatic methods.

Clinical information, nomograms, and equations on dosage adjustment and drug clearance are usually based on Cl_{Cr}.

Creatinine is a metabolic by-product of muscle breakdown, and its production rate is determined by the patient's muscle mass. Differences in muscle mass are observed between genders and various age groups. Creatinine production is relatively constant in any given patient and, once produced, is excreted almost entirely by glomerular filtration. Hence, Cl_{Cr} is a reasonable measure of glomerular filtration. At steady state, the rate of creatinine production equals the rate of creatinine excretion. Therefore, by measuring the creatinine concentration one can estimate the Cl_{Cr}.

$$Cl_{Cr} = \frac{\text{Rate of Production}}{\text{Plasma Concentration}} \qquad \textbf{(Eq. 24)}$$

Adult Creatinine Clearance

The calculation of Cl_{Cr} from serum creatinine concentrations (SrCr) is described in greater detail in **Basic Clinical Pharmacokinetics**, 3rd ed.[1] We recommend the Cockcroft and Gault approach to estimate Cl_{Cr} since it accounts for differences in gender, weight, and age. This method assumes SrCr is at steady state, the weight included in the formula reflects normal muscle mass, and the patient's age is >18 yr.

$$\begin{matrix} Cl_{Cr} \text{ for Males} \\ \text{(mL/min)} \end{matrix} = \frac{(140 - \text{Age})(\text{Weight in kg})}{(72)(SrCr_{ss})} \qquad \textbf{(Eq. 25)}$$
(Eq 63, pg 95)

$$\begin{matrix} Cl_{Cr} \text{ for Females} \\ \text{(mL/min)} \end{matrix} = (0.85)\frac{(140 - \text{Age})(\text{Weight in kg})}{(72)(SrCr_{ss})} \qquad \textbf{(Eq. 26)}$$
(Eq 64, pg 95)

Total body weight (TBW) may be used in the above equations for patients at their ideal body weight (IBW) or <20% above their IBW. Actual body weight should be used in patients who are < their IBW. In patients >20% above their IBW, IBW can be estimated as follows:

$$\text{IBW for Males in kg} = 50 + (2.3)(\text{Height in Inches} > 60) \qquad \textbf{(Eq. 27)}$$

(Eq 65, pg 96)

$$\text{IBW for Females in kg} = 45 + (2.3)(\text{Height in Inches} > 60) \qquad \textbf{(Eq. 28)}$$

(Eq 66, pg 96)

Pediatric Creatinine Clearance

The Cl_{Cr} in pediatric patients (age 1–18 yr) can be estimated (normalized to 70 kg or 1.73 m²) with the following equation:

$$\text{Cl}_{Cr} \text{ for Children (mL/min/1.73 m}^2\text{)} = \frac{(0.48)(\text{Height in cm})}{\text{SrCr}_{ss}} \qquad \textbf{(Eq. 29)}$$

(Eq 68, pg 98)

To normalize the value obtained from the above equation to the patient's actual Cl_{Cr}, the following equation may be used. Body surface area (BSA) can be determined by use of the nomogram in Appendix I.

$$\text{Cl}_{Cr} \text{ for Children (mL/min)} = (\text{Cl}_{Cr} \text{ mL/min/1.73 m}^2)\left(\frac{\text{BSA}}{1.73 \text{ m}^2}\right) \qquad \textbf{(Eq. 30)}$$

(Eq 69, pg 98)

Nonsteady-State Creatinine

The following equation can be used in situations when creatinine concentrations are increasing or decreasing in both adult and pediatric patients. The daily production of creatinine can be calculated from Table 1. The patient's serum creatinine concentrations (SrCr) should be expressed in mg/L; therefore, the usual concentrations reported by clinical laboratories in mg/dL should be multiplied by a factor of 10.

$$\frac{Cl_{Cr}}{(L/day)} = \frac{\left[\begin{array}{c}\text{Daily Production of}\\ \text{Creatinine in mg}\end{array}\right] - \left[\dfrac{(SrCr_2 - SrCr_1)(Vd_{Cr})}{t}\right]}{SrCr_2}$$

(Eq. 31)
(Eq 70, pg 99)

where: Vd of Creatinine (Vd_{Cr}) = 0.5 L/kg

t = time interval between SrCr concentrations

For a more thorough discussion of this equation refer to **Basic Clinical Pharmacokinetics**, 3rd ed.[1]

Notes:

Table 1	Expected Daily Creatinine Production for Males[a]
Age (yr)	Daily Creatinine Production (mg/kg/day)
20–29	24
30–39	22
40–49	20
50–59	19
60–69	17
70–79	14
80–89	12
90–99	9

[a]For females, multiply the expected creatinine production by 0.85.

24-Hour Urine Collections

Cl_{Cr} can be more directly assessed by use of 24-hr urine collections in conjunction with SrCr measurements. With this approach, the following basic equation is utilized:

$$\frac{Cl_{Cr}}{(mL/min)} = \frac{(u * V/p)}{1440}$$

where: u = Urine creatinine concentration (mg/dL)

V = Urine volume

p = Average plasma creatinine concentration (mg/dL)

1440 = # of min/24 hr

Determining the Cl_{Cr} by measuring the amount of creatinine in a 24-hr urine collection is not without problems. A voided urine sample can be missed or lost during the 24-hr period which results in underestimation of Cl_{Cr}; alternatively, urine may be collected for more than 24 hr, in which case the Cl_{Cr} will be greater than expected. Even under the best of conditions, 24-hr collections should be evaluated critically. The expected amount of creatinine production should be estimated from Table 1 and compared to the concentration reported by the laboratory (u * V). If the expected production of creatinine differs significantly (± 2 S.D.) from the collected creatinine, the sample should be viewed as possibly incomplete or excessive. When the reported creatinine production is outside this range, or the clinical presentation is not consistent with creatinine production (e.g., creatinine production may be decreased in a cachectic individual), the Cl_{Cr} obtained by this method is not used.

References

1. Winter ME. Basic Clinical Pharmacokinetics, 3rd ed. Vancouver: Applied Therapeutics; 1994.93–103.

2. Rowland M, Tozer T. Clinical Pharmacokinetics, Concepts and Applications, 2nd ed. Philadelphia: Lea and Febiger; 1989:192.

Notes:

Dialysis

All forms of dialysis potentially can alter the pharmacokinetic disposition of medications. Dialysis methods have proliferated over the past two decades and now include hemodialysis, peritoneal dialysis, hemoperfusion, hemofiltration, and others. The guidelines described in this chapter apply to hemodialysis; however, these are generalizations and may not hold true for all medications in all situations. Additional factors such as brand and type of hemodialysis filter and different blood flow rates during the procedure can confound the clinician's assessment. Several characteristics of a drug can be analyzed to determine whether its pharmacokinetic disposition is likely to be significantly altered by hemodialysis.

Volume of Distribution (Vd)

When volume of distribution (Vd)/the free fraction (α) exceeds 250 L, the drug probably will not be dialyzed to a significant degree. As the Vd increases and α decreases, less drug is available for filtration (i.e., the drug is extensively tissue-bound with very little drug in the plasma compartment available for dialysis).

Clearance (Cl)

When Cl exceeds 500 mL/min, the drug probably will not be dialyzed to a significant degree. Most drugs that are cleared by hemodialysis have dialysis clearances (Cl_{dial}) in the range of 5–50 mL. This low Cl will not significantly add to patient clearances (Cl_{pat}) that are >500 mL/min.

Half-Life (t½)

If t½ is short (i.e., 1–3 hr), the drug may be dialyzed to a significant degree. However, the consequences usually will be minimal because even under non-dialysis conditions very little drug will remain at the end of the dosing interval (τ). Since medications with very short t½s do not tend to significantly accumulate when dosed intermittently, it is not likely that dosage alterations will be required with the addition of hemodialysis. In some cases the practitioner may elect to administer the usual dose timed so that it is given after dialysis. In the evaluation of the t½ factor, the patient's estimated t½ must be evaluated rather than the "normal" literature-derived t½.

Molecular Weight

If the drug's molecular weight >1200, it probably will not be dialyzed to a significant degree.

If an assessment of the above four factors suggests that a drug's clearance from dialysis may be significant, then a thorough literature search for actual Cl_{dial} values may be appropriate. When an actual Cl_{dial} value can be obtained from the literature, the following equation can be used to determine the significance of Cl_{dial} in a given patient.

$$t\tfrac{1}{2} \text{ during Hemodialysis} = \frac{(0.693)(Vd)}{(Cl_{pat} + Cl_{dial})} \quad \text{(Eq 83, pg 109)}$$

When t½ during dialysis approaches or is shorter than the duration of dialysis, the contribution of Cl_{dial} to Cl_{pat} can be significant and may warrant a dose or τ adjustment.

The following two models can be used to assess drug concentrations in patients undergoing hemodialysis. Model I is appropriate when τ is much shorter than t½. (See Figure 7 on page 43.) In this situation very little drug is lost between doses. Model II is appropriate to use when $\tau > t\frac{1}{2}$ and variations in peak to trough concentrations are significant during the interval. (See Figure 8 on page 44.) For more information concerning these models, please refer to **Basic Clinical Pharmacokinetics,** 3rd ed.[1]

Model I Equations

$$\text{Cpss ave} = \frac{(S)(F)(Dose/\tau)}{Cl_{pat}} \qquad \text{(Eq 73, pg 104)}$$

$$\text{Dose} = \frac{(\text{Cpss ave})(Cl_{pat})(\tau)}{(S)(F)} \qquad \text{(Eq 74, pg 104)}$$

Postdialysis
Replacement $= (Vd)(\text{Cpss ave})\left(1 - e^{-\left(\frac{Cl_{pat} + Cl_{dial}}{Vd}\right)(T_d)}\right)$
Dose

(Eq 76, pg 105)

$$= \begin{bmatrix} \text{Amount of Drug} \\ \text{in the Body} \\ \text{Prior to Dialysis} \end{bmatrix} \begin{bmatrix} \text{Fraction of Drug} \\ \text{Lost During Dialysis} \end{bmatrix}$$

(Eq 75, pg 104)

$$= (Vd)(\text{Cpss ave})\left(1 - e^{-(K_{dial})(T_d)}\right)$$

(Eq 77, pg 105)

where: T_d = time dialysis

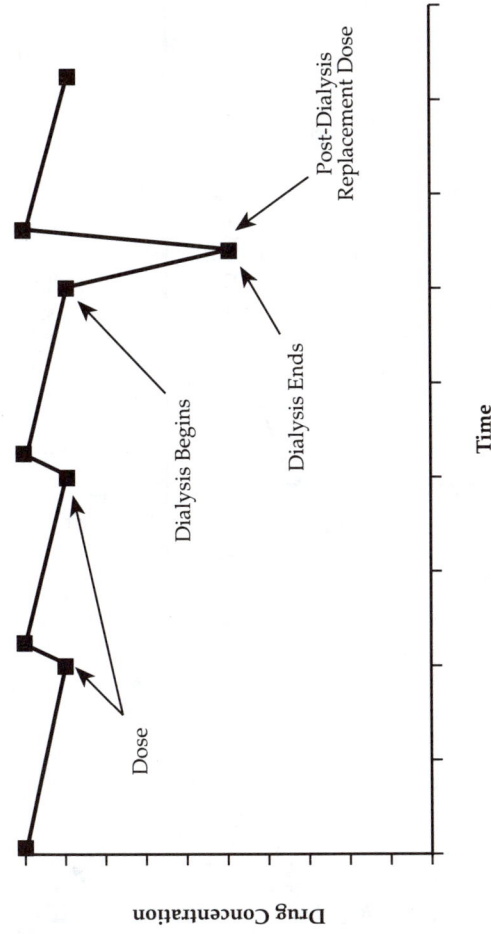

Figure 7. Model I. Note that the peak to trough variation is small and the concentration at any time during the interval (nondialysis interval) may be viewed as a Cpss ave concentration.

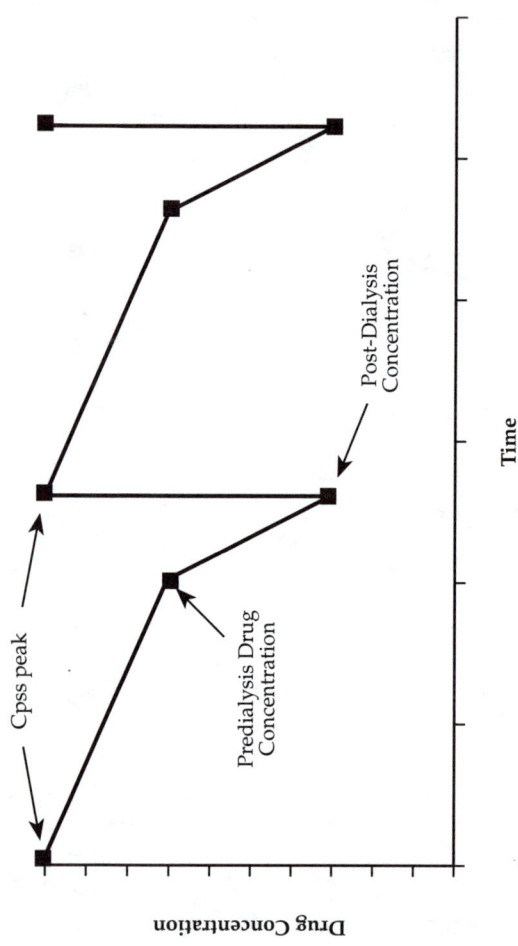

Figure 8. Model II.

Model II Equations

$$\begin{array}{c}\text{Predialysis}\\\text{Drug Concentration}\end{array} = \text{Cpss max}\left(e^{-\frac{Cl_{pat}}{Vd}(t_1)}\right) \quad \text{(Eq 80, pg 107)}$$

$$\begin{array}{c}\text{Postdialysis}\\\text{Drug Concentration}\end{array} = \left(\begin{array}{c}\text{Predialysis}\\\text{Drug}\\\text{Concentration}\end{array}\right)\left(e^{-\left(\frac{Cl_{pat} + Cl_{dial}}{Vd}\right)(T_d)}\right)$$

$$\text{(Eq 81, pg 107)}$$

$$\begin{array}{c}\text{Postdialysis}\\\text{Replacement Dose}\end{array} = (Vd)(\text{Cpss max})$$
$$\left(1 - \left[\left(e^{-\frac{Cl_{pat}}{Vd}(t_1)}\right)\left(e^{-\left(\frac{Cl_{pat} + Cl_{dial}}{Vd}\right)(T_d)}\right)\right]\right)$$

$$\text{(Eq 78, pg 105)}$$

$$= (Vd)(\text{Cpss max})\left(1 - \left[\left(e^{-(Kd_{pat})(t_1)}\right)\left(e^{-(K_{dial})(T_d)}\right)\right]\right)$$

$$\text{(Eq 79, pg 105)}$$

References

1. Winter ME. Basic Clinical Pharmacokinetics, 3rd ed. Vancouver: Applied Therapeutics; 1994:104–118.

Aminoglycosides 1

(Gentamicin, Tobramycin, Amikacin)

The aminoglycoside antibiotics have excellent activity against aerobic gram-negative organisms including *Pseudomonas aeruginosa*. They frequently are used, either alone or in combination with other agents, to treat bacteremia, pneumonia, complicated urinary tract infections, burn wounds, osteomyelitis, peritonitis, and other serious gram-negative infections. Although aminoglycoside-induced nephrotoxicity and ototoxicity are of concern, appropriate dosing and adequate monitoring greatly diminish the incidence of these adverse effects. Well described correlations between plasma levels, efficacy, and toxicity have placed the aminoglycosides at the top of the list for drugs that are monitored pharmacokinetically.

The aminoglycosides elicit their bactericidal effect by inhibiting bacterial protein synthesis at the level of the 30S ribosome. The development of resistance to aminoglycosides typically involves inactivation by enzymes such as adenylase (gentamicin and tobramycin) and acetylase (amikacin). Because inactivation occurs by different enzymes, organisms resistant to gentamicin or tobramycin may still be susceptible to amikacin.

The monobactam, aztreonam (Azactam), has a spectrum of activity similar to the aminoglycosides without the apparent risk of nephrotoxicity. Aztreonam should not be thought of as a replacement for aminoglycosides, but as an alternative for patients who are at risk for aminoglycoside-induced nephrotoxicity (i.e., the elderly, patients with underlying renal disease).

Dose

Aminoglycosides are administered intermittently by one of the following routes: intravenous, intramuscular, intraventricular [central nervous system (CNS) infections], or intrathecal (CNS infections). Because aminoglycosides are not readily distributed into adipose tissue, dosing should be based upon ideal body weight (IBW) rather than actual body weight.

Loading Dose

> ➪ Often utilized in serious infections.

> ➪ Based upon desired Cp, an estimate of the patient's volume of distribution (Vd), and severity of infection.

> ➪ *General guidelines:*

>> □ gentamicin and tobramycin: 1–2 mg/kg

>> □ amikacin: 5–7 mg/kg

>> □ *note:* the upper limit may be even higher in immunocompromised septic patients

Maintenance Dose

Initial

> ➪ Should consider patient's estimated clearance (Cl) and the severity of the infection.

> ➪ *General guidelines:*

>> □ gentamicin and tobramycin: usually does not exceed 6 mg/kg/day

>> □ amikacin: usually does not exceed 15 mg/kg/day

⇨ Young patients and patients with cystic fibrosis typically require short dosage intervals due to enhanced Cl.

□ administer in divided doses based on patient's renal function.

Maintenance regimen

⇨ "Fine-tuned" after obtaining patient-specific plasma concentration information.

⇨ Patient-specific parameters (t½, Cl, and Vd) can be calculated once the appropriate data are collected.

⇨ See Useful Pharmacokinetic Equations: Calculations of Pharmacokinetic Parameters Based Upon Patient-Specific Parameters on page 56.

Dosing Methods and Nomograms

⇨ The more specific information that is incorporated in the regimen, the more accurate the recommendation.

⇨ *Empiric:* 80 mg Q 8 hr (gentamicin, tobramycin).

⇨ *Based upon body weight:*

□ 3–6 mg/kg/day or 1–2 mg/kg/dose (gentamicin, tobramycin).

□ 15–20 mg/kg/day or 5–7 mg/kg/dose (amikacin).[7]

⇨ *Rule of eights:* 1–1.6 mg/kg Q (8 hr × SrCr) (gentamicin, tobramycin).[3]

⇨ *Nomograms:* See Figures 1.1 and 1.2.

□ created to assist in calculating dosage regimens

□ limitations:
  ○ imperfect correlation between creatinine and aminoglycoside Cl
  ○ developed based upon a small number of patients (20–30)
  ○ do not take into consideration potential changes in distribution volume
  ○ should only be used as a rough estimate in noncritically ill patients

Therapeutic & Toxic Range

⇨ Desired plasma concentrations will depend upon the type and severity of the infection and the specific aminoglycoside agent utilized.

⇨ Toxicity associated with aminoglycosides has not been clearly correlated with specific plasma concentrations. However, trough concentrations that are persistently >2 mg/L are associated with ototoxicity as well as nephrotoxicity (↑ SrCr and ↓ Cl_{Cr}). In the critical care setting, however, it often is difficult to determine whether the increased trough concentration is the result of or the cause of the nephrotoxicity.

⇨ Toxicity is likely to be correlated with the area under the concentration-time curve (AUC) rather than a single elevated peak or trough concentration.

Aminoglycoside Dosing Chart

1. Select loading dose in mg/kg (IBW) to provide peak plasma levels in range listed below for desired aminoglycoside.

Aminoglycoside	Usual Loading Doses	Expected Peak Plasma Levels
Tobramycin Gentamicin	1.5–2.0 mg/kg	4–10 µg/mL
Amikacin Kanamycin	5.0–7.5 mg/kg	15–30 µg/mL

2. Select maintenance dose (as percentage of chosen loading dose) to continue peak plasma levels indicated above according to desired dosing interval and the patient's corrected creatinine clearance[a]

Figure 1.1. Hull-Sarubbi dosage nomogram. Reprinted with permission from reference 5.

**Percentage of Loading Dose Required
For Dosage Interval Selected**

Cl_{Cr} (cor)[b] (mL/min)	$t\frac{1}{2}$c (hr)	8 hr (%)	12 hr (%)	24 hr (%)
90	3.1	84	—	—
80	3.4	80	91	—
70	3.9	76	88	—
60	4.5	71	84	—
50	5.3	65	79	92
40	6.5	57	72	86
30	8.4	48	63	81
25	9.9	43	57	75
20	11.9	37	50	70
17	13.6	33	46	67
15	15.1	31	42	61
12	17.9	27	37	56
10	20.4	24	34	47
7	25.9	19	28	41
5	31.5	16	23	30
2	46.8	11	16	30
0	69.3	8	11	21

[a] Calculate corrected creatinine clearance [Cl_{Cr} (cor)] as:

Cl_{Cr} (cor) male = (140–age)/serum creatinine Cl_{Cr} (cor) female = 0.85 × Cl_{Cr} (cor) male

[b] Dosing for patients with Cl_{Cr} (cor) <10 mL/min should be assisted by measured plasma levels.

[c] Alternatively, ½ of the chosen loading dose may be given at an interval approximately equal to the estimated $t\frac{1}{2}$.

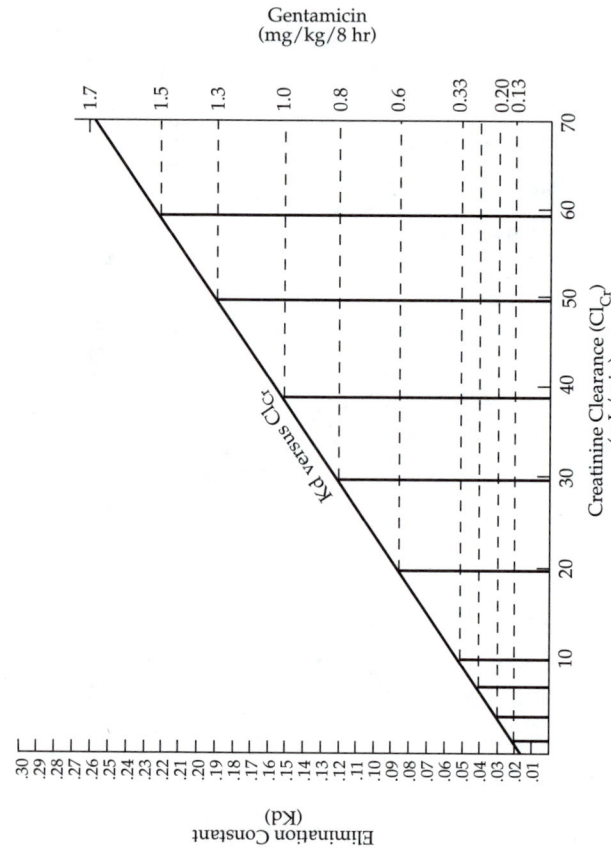

Figure 1.2. Chan dosage nomogram for patients with renal failure. Reprinted with permission from reference 4.

⇨ *Desired plasma concentrations:*

Type of Infection	Gentamicin & Tobramycin		Amikacin	
	peaks (mg/L)	troughs (mg/L)	peaks (mg/L)	troughs (mg/L)
Severe to life-threatening	8–10	<2	25–32	4–8
Moderate to mild	6–8	<2	20–25	2–4
Urinary tract	4–6	<2	15–20	2–4

Pharmacokinetic Parameters

Bioavailability (F)

⇨ Oral absorption is minimal (1%–4%).

⇨ Absorption may be erratic and incomplete after intramuscular (IM) administration; avoid IM in critically ill patients with reduced skeletal muscle perfusion or decreased muscle mass.

⇨ Peak plasma concentrations occur 30–120 min after IM injections (average: 60 min).

Volume of Distribution (Vd)

⇨ Rapidly and widely distributed, primarily in extracellular fluid (ECF).

⇨ Water soluble; therefore, little is distributed into adipose tissue (base dose on IBW).

⇨ Poor penetration into cerebral spinal fluid (CSF); utilize intrathecal or intraventricular routes.

⇨ Slight distribution phase exists (5–15 min); clinically insignificant if dose is administered over 30–60 min.

⇨ Vd = 0.25 L/kg (0.15–0.35 L/kg).

⇨ *Factors influencing Vd:*

- □ hydration status (increase or decrease)

- □ congestive heart failure (CHF) increased Vd initially; after diuresis Vd may decrease to normal

- □ sepsis increased initially during hydration; decrease after stabilization

- □ severe edema (increase)

- □ burn patients increase initially; after diuresis Vd will drop *sharply*

- □ neonates (increase — 0.5 L/kg)

- □ ascites (increase)

⇨ Critically important to closely monitor patients with changing clinical status.

Clearance (Cl) & Half-Life (t½)

⇨ 95% of elimination is by kidneys.

⇨ Slight nonrenal Cl; clinically insignificant except in patients with chronic renal impairment.

⇨ Creatinine clearance (Cl_{Cr}) can be used as a rough estimate of aminoglycoside Cl.

⇨ Normal t½ = 1.5–3 hr.

⇨ *Factors influencing Cl:*

- □ reduced renal function (↓ Cl)

- □ burn patients (↑ Cl)

□ stress and trauma (↑ Cl)

□ patients with cystic fibrosis (↑ Cl)

Useful Pharmacokinetic Equations

Estimating Initial Pharmacokinetic Parameters

Volume of distribution (L)

$$Vd = 0.25 \text{ L/kg (based upon IBW)}$$

Drug clearance (L/hr)

⇨ Use Cl_{Cr} as an estimate of aminoglycoside Cl.

$$\frac{Cl_{Cr} \text{ for Males}}{\text{(mL/min)}} = \frac{(140 - \text{Age})(\text{Weight based upon IBW})}{(72)(SrCr_{ss})}$$

(Eq 63, pg 95)

$$\frac{Cl_{Cr} \text{ for Females}}{\text{(mL/min)}} = 0.85 \, (Cl_{Cr} \text{ for Males})$$

(Eq 64, pg 95)

⇨ Convert units from mL/min to L/hr.

$$\frac{Cl_{Cr}}{\text{(L/hr)}} = \left(\frac{Cl_{Cr}}{\text{in mL/min}}\right)\left(\frac{1L}{1000 \text{ mL}}\right)\left(\frac{60 \text{ min}}{1 \text{ mL}}\right)$$

Elimination rate constant (hr⁻¹) & half-life (hr)

$$\frac{Kd}{(hr^{-1})} = \frac{Cl \text{ (in L/hr)}}{Vd \text{ (in L)}}$$

(Eq 27, pg 41)

$$\frac{t^{1/2}}{\text{(hr)}} = \frac{0.693}{Kd}$$

(Eq 31, pg 43)

Determining an Initial Dosage Regimen

Dosage interval (hr)

$$\tau \approx 3 \times \text{estimated } t^{1/2}$$

⇨ Round to convenient intervals of 6, 8, 12, 24 hr.

Dosage calculation (mg)

$$\text{Dose} = \frac{Cpss_2(1 - e^{-Kd\tau})}{\dfrac{(S)(F/t_{in})}{Cl}(1 - e^{-Kdt_{in}})(e^{-Kdt_2})}$$

where: t_{in} = Time of infusion
t_2 = Time from end of infusion to time to sample

Expected trough concentration (or Cp at any given time t)

$$Cp_t = (Cp^0)(e^{-(Kdt)})$$

where: Cp_t = Expected concentration at time (t)
after the initial concentration (Cp^0)

Calculations of Pharmacokinetic Parameters
Based Upon Patient-Specific Concentration Data

Elimination rate constant (hr⁻¹) and half-life (hr)

$$Kd = \frac{\ln\left(\dfrac{Cp_1}{Cp_2}\right)}{(t_1 - t_2)}$$

$$t^{1/2} = \frac{0.693}{Kd} \qquad \text{(Eq 31, pg 43)}$$

Drug clearance (L/hr)

$$Cl = \frac{\dfrac{(S)(F)(Dose/t_{in})}{Cpss_2} (1 - e^{-Kdt_{in}})}{(1 - e^{-Kd\tau})} (e^{-Kdt_2})$$

(Eq 1.7, pg 152)

Volume of distribution (L)

$$Vd = \frac{Cl(L/hr)}{Kd(hr^{-1})}$$

(Eq 1.8, pg 153)

⇨ Always assess the "believability" of the calculated parameters before using them to calculate a regimen.

⇨ "Fine-tune" the dosage regimen by calculating a new maintenance dose based upon the patient-specific parameters:

$$\frac{Dose}{(mg)} = \frac{Cpss_2 (1 - e^{-Kd\tau})}{\dfrac{(S)(F/t_{in})}{Cl} (1 - e^{-Kdt_{in}})(e^{-Kdt_2})}$$

Expected concentration at a given time (t_2)

$$Cpss_2 = \frac{\dfrac{(S)(F)(Dose/t_{in})}{Cl} (1 - e^{-Kdt_{in}})}{(1 - e^{-Kd\tau})} (e^{-Kdt_2})$$

⇨ To calculate true Cpss max (directly at the end of the infusion), $t_2 = 0$ and e^{-Kdt_2} is dropped.

⇨ To calculate true Cpss min (just before the next dose), $t_2 = (\tau - t_{in})$.

Serum Sampling Strategies

Two general strategies exist for obtaining aminoglycoside plasma concentrations: a peak and trough study once the patient has reached steady state or a first-dose kinetic study.

⇨ Steady-state conditions are achieved after ≈3–5 t½s.

⇨ Renal and fluid status must remain stable and strict adherence to the dosing schedule must be maintained.

⇨ *Peak and trough study.* (See Figure 1.3.)

   □ most frequently used sampling strategy

   □ steady-state plasma concentrations are obtained just before the dose (trough) and 30–60 min after the end of the infusion period (peak)

   □ used mostly in patients with less severe infections and shorter t½s (turn-around time is short)

   □ the majority of follow-up pharmacokinetic studies use peak and trough evaluations

⇨ *First-dose study.* (See Figure 1.4.)

   □ a series of plasma concentrations are obtained after the initial dose

      ○ 1) 30–60 min after the end of the infusion

      ○ 2) somewhere in between 1 and 3

      ○ 3) 1½–2 times the estimated t½

   □ used in situations where aggressive, prompt therapy is required or it is not feasible to wait for steady-state conditions

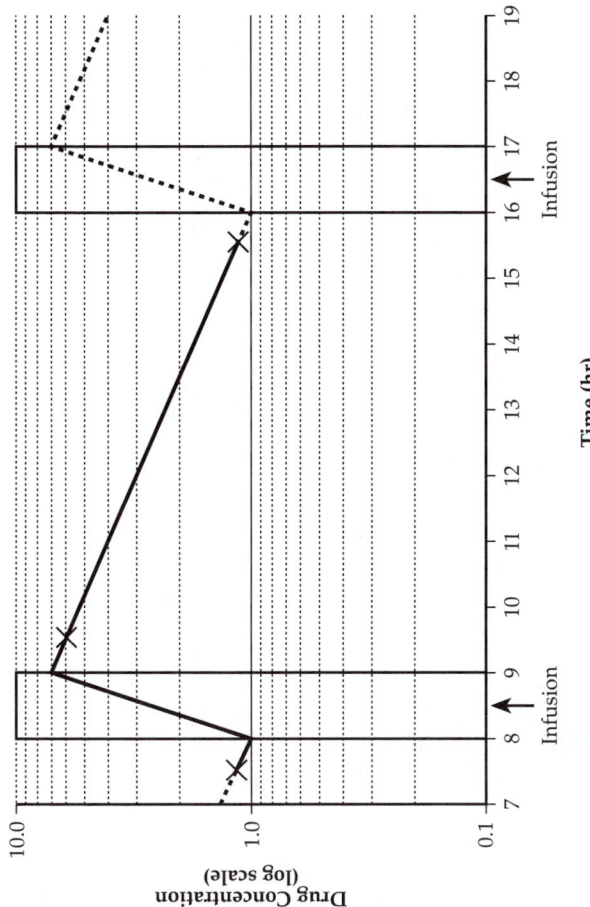

Figure 1.3. Peak and trough study.

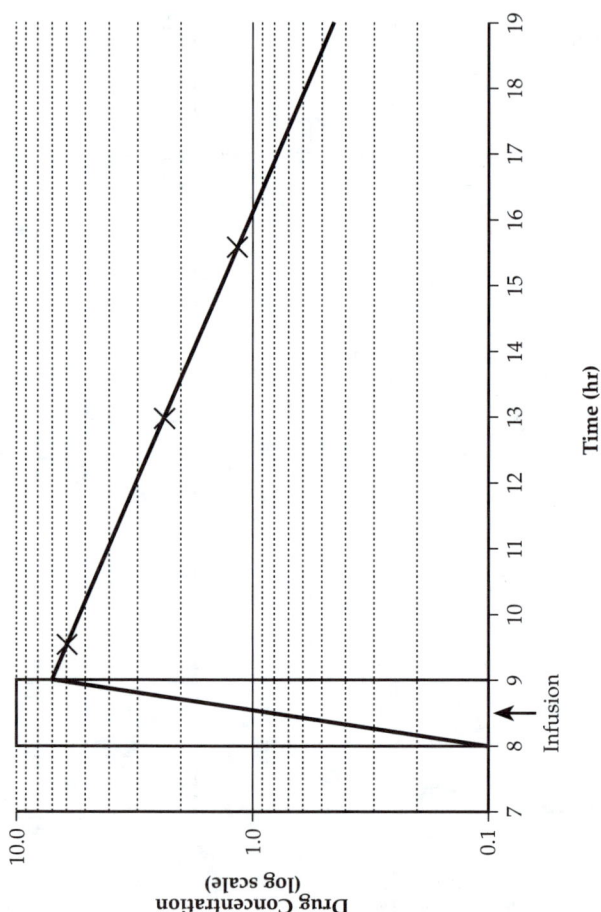

Figure 1.4. First dose study.

         □ most appropriate in the elderly, critically ill, or patients with compromised renal function

Dialyzability

Hemodialysis

    ⇨ Significantly removes aminoglycosides.

    ⇨ Specific removal rate depends on flow rate, dialysis membrane utilized, and total duration of the dialysis run.

    ⇨ Supplemental doses often are required after dialysis.

    ⇨ Separate clearance rates (Cl_{pat} and Cl_{dial}) can also be used to predict dosage requirements.[1]

Peritoneal

    ⇨ Clearance of aminoglycosides can be enhanced.

    ⇨ The extent and efficiency of the removal is less than with hemodialysis.

    ⇨ Extent depends upon peritoneal dialysate dwell time.

Monitoring Parameters

Subjective

    ⇨ Improvement in patient well being.

    ⇨ Decreased hearing ability or balance problems.

Objective

⇨ Aminoglycoside plasma concentrations.

⇨ Microbiology cultures.

⇨ White blood cell (WBC) count and differential.

⇨ Temperature (afebrile).

⇨ BUN/SrCr.

⇨ Urinary output (I/O).

⇨ Urinalysis.

Drug Interactions

⇨ *Anti-pseudomonal penicillins* (carbenicillin, ticarcillin, mezlocillin, azlocillin, piperacillin)

  □ *In vitro* inactivation of aminoglycosides (primarily gentamicin and tobramycin) can occur in the presence of semi-synthetic penicillins.

  □ This interaction is dependent upon the concentration of agents, as well as the duration of exposure and temperature; it occurs most often in patients with significant renal impairment.

  □ To avoid potential interactions, serum samples from patients receiving both antibiotics should be processed promptly or placed on ice to minimize the interaction.

⇨ *Amphotericin B* enhances aminoglycoside toxicity.

⇨ *Vancomycin* enhances aminoglycoside toxicity.

⇨ *Diuretics (dehydration)* enhance aminoglycoside toxicity.

⇨ *Heparin,* in high concentrations, may inactivate aminoglycosides.

Special Considerations

Potential for Once-Daily Dosing

⇨ Administering the total daily aminoglycoside dose as a single rather than intermittent dose may prove more effective with less risk for toxicity.

⇨ This has only been established in patients who are not neutropenic or severely immunosuppressed.

⇨ Studies involving single-dose aminoglycoside therapy use a variety of dosage regimens.[6]

⇨ Peak concentrations are significantly greater than with traditional regimens.

⇨ Trough concentrations tend to fall below 1.0 mg/L before the subsequent dose.

⇨ The post-antibiotic effect (PAE) may contribute to the continued bacterial killing despite concentrations below the minimum inhibitory concentration (MIC) toward the end of the 24-hr dosing interval.

⇨ This dosing approach could change the well-established and commonly-practiced methods for dosing and monitoring aminoglycosides.

⇨ Additional clinical trials are necessary to fully characterize the role of once-daily aminoglycoside dosing.

References

1. Winter ME. Basic Clinical Pharmacokinetics. 3rd ed. Vancouver: Applied Therapeutics; 1994:128–176.

2. Zaske DE. Aminoglycosides. In: Evans WE et al, eds. Applied Pharmacokinetics: Principles of Therapeutic Drug Monitoring. 3rd ed. Vancouver: Applied Therapeutics; 1992:14-1–14-47.

3. Zaske DE et al. Aminoglycosides. In: Taylor WT, Diers-Caviness MH, eds. A Textbook for the Clinical Application of Therapeutic Drug Monitoring. Irving, TX: Abbott Laboratories Diagnostic Division; 1986:285–320.

4. Chan RA et al. Gentamicin therapy in renal failure: a nomogram for dosage. Ann Intern Med. 1972;76:773–778.

5. Sarubbi FA, Hull JH. Amikacin serum concentrations: prediction of levels and dosage guidelines. Ann Intern Med. 1978; 89:612–618.

6. Gilbert DN. Once-daily aminoglycoside therapy. Antimicrob Agents Chemother. 1991;35:399–405.

7. Barriere SL, Dudley MN. Aminoglycosides. In: Knoben JE. Anderson PO, eds. Handbook of Clinical Drug Data. 7th ed. Hamilton, IL: Drug Intelligence Publications; 1993:338.

Notes:

Carbamazepine 2

Carbamazepine is an anticonvulsant effective in the management of generalized tonic-clonic seizures and complex, partial seizures. It also is effective in the management of patients with trigeminal neuralgias (tic douloureux) and other neurological disorders. Carbamazepine has the unique capability of inducing its own metabolism (auto-induction). When carbamazepine is added to an existing regimen of anticonvulsants, it is likely that the metabolism of these agents will also be induced, and dosages may need to be adjusted. A narrow therapeutic index and several concentration-dependent toxicities make plasma concentration monitoring an important component of carbamazepine therapy.

Dose

Loading Dose

⇨ The auto-induction capability of carbamazepine requires therapy to be initiated at low doses and gradually increased as auto-induction takes effect.

⇨ Loading dose should *NOT* be administered to avoid high plasma concentrations *and the associated toxicity.*

Maintenance Dose

⇨ Steady-state maintenance dose is calculated based upon the patient's Cl and the desired plasma concentration.

⇨ Therapy is usually initiated as either 100 or 200 mg BID.

⇨ Dose is gradually titrated upward by 100–200 mg increments at 1–2 week intervals or as tolerated.

- ☐ titration can be more aggressive in patients already taking an enzyme-inducing agent
- ☐ children (6–12 yr) are started at 100 mg BID and increased by 100 mg increments

⇨ Continue to increase dose until seizures are controlled, toxicity develops, or the full steady-state daily dose is reached.

⇨ Daily doses >800 mg should be divided into 3 or 4 equal doses to minimize toxicity.

⇨ After desired effect is reached adjust regimen to the minimum effective dose.

⇨ Abrupt withdrawal of carbamazepine may cause significant seizures and possibly, status epilepticus.

⇨ *General dosing guidelines:*

- ☐ adults: 10–20 mg/kg/day
- ☐ children ages 6–12: 20–30 mg/kg/day

Therapeutic & Toxic Range

⇨ A fair degree of variation exists in the therapeutic range of carbamazepine: 4–12 mg/L.

⇨ Side effects tend to correlate with high plasma concentrations.

- ☐ avoid by gradually titrating dosage upward
- ☐ consider giving a smaller dose more frequently to avoid high concentrations

⇨ Dose-related toxicities include nystagmus, sedation, ataxia, blurred vision, and headache.

  □ mild toxicity: >4 mg/L

  □ more severe toxicity: >8–10 mg/L

⇨ Serious idiosyncratic toxicities are rare and include nondose-dependent aplastic anemia, leukopenia, and Stevens-Johnson syndrome.

Pharmacokinetic Parameters

Bioavailability (F)

⇨ Only available as oral products.

  □ tablets: 100 and 200 mg

  □ oral suspension: 100 mg/5 mL

⇨ Bioavailability varies substantially: average 80% (70%–100%).

⇨ Not formulated as a salt; therefore, S = 1.0 (100%).

⇨ Absorption from the GI tract is very slow and variable.

  □ food may enhance (i.e., increase) absorption

  □ changes in the GI transit time also affect absorption

⇨ Plasma concentrations usually peak about 6 hr (range: 2–24 hr) after a dose.

Volume of Distribution (Vd)

⇨ Widely distributed. Vd = 1.4 L/kg (range: 0.8–1.9 L/kg).

⇨ 70%–80% of carbamazepine is bound to protein (primarily albumin).

⇨ CSF:serum ratio = 0.15–0.30 (resembles the fraction unbound).

   □ similar amount is distributed in saliva

   □ monitoring salivary concentrations may provide an estimate of CSF concentrations

⇨ Displacement of carbamazepine by other drugs does not appear to be a problem.

   □ valproic acid may slightly increase carbamazepine plasma concentrations

Clearance (Cl) & Half-Life (t½)

⇨ Primary route of elimination is hepatic metabolism.

⇨ Epoxide metabolite plays a role in activity of carbamazepine.

⇨ Carbamazepine has a low extraction ratio (ER = 0.20).

⇨ Auto-induction.

   □ rate of carbamazepine Cl will increase over time and as the dose increases (see Serum Sampling Strategies on page 69)

   □ carbamazepine also increases Cl of other agents by cross-induction

⇨ Average steady-state Cl = 0.064 L/hr/kg (takes into account auto-induction).

⇨ *Factors that influence carbamazepine Cl:*

   □ as age increases, Cl decreases and higher plasma concentrations are achieved

   □ concurrent use of enzyme inducers increases clearance

- □ young children treated with multiple anticonvulsants will have the most rapid carbamazepine Cl

⇨ t½ will vary based on the extent of auto-induction present:

- □ t½ = 30–35 hr (initially) before auto-induction
- □ t½ = 15 hr (steady state); takes into consideration auto-induction

Useful Pharmacokinetic Equations

Oral Maintenance Dose

$$\frac{\text{Maintenance Dose}}{\text{(mg/day)}} = \frac{(\text{Cl})(\text{Cpss ave})(\tau)}{(\text{S})(\text{F})} \qquad \text{(Eq 16, pg 28)}$$

Serum Sampling Strategies

⇨ Steady-state conditions are reached after 3 days of an unchanged carbamazepine regimen. Dosing regimen adjustments will require time to reach a new steady state.

⇨ Samples should be obtained just before the next dose (trough) to avoid effects of the slow absorption rate.

⇨ Any increase in dose will result in a *less than proportional* increase in plasma concentration due to auto-induction.

⇨ Plasma concentrations are useful in affirming therapeutic effect or suspected toxicity.

⇨ Plasma concentrations should be monitored when other anticonvulsant agents are added or deleted.

□ serum levels for all drugs should be evaluated

□ consider the appropriate sampling time for each specific anticonvulsant

Dialyzability

Hemodialysis & Peritoneal:

⇨ It is unclear whether hemodialysis or peritoneal dialysis removes carbamazepine.

Monitoring Parameters

Subjective

⇨ Decreased mentation, complaints of headache.

⇨ Nystagmus.

⇨ Seizure control or seizure frequency.

⇨ Compliance.

Objective

⇨ Serum carbamazepine.

⇨ White blood cell (WBC) count with differential.

⇨ Platelets.

⇨ Electroencephalogram (EEG).

⇨ BUN/SrCr.

⇨ Liver function tests (LFTs).

Drug Interactions

⇨ Can interact with many drugs because of hepatic enzyme induction.

Table 2.1	Carbamazepine Drug Interactions
Drugs that ↓ Carbamazepine Cl	*Carbamazepine will ↑Cl of*
Verapamil	Warfarin
Erythromycin	Theophylline
Propoxyphene	Other anticonvulsants
Cimetidine	Oral contraceptives

Special Considerations

⇨ The *primary goal* of treating any seizure disorder is to achieve the best seizure control possible with the smallest dose of anticonvulsant to minimize the potential for adverse events.

⇨ *Clinical response.* The large degree of pharmacokinetic variability between and within patients makes it very difficult to pinpoint an effective therapeutic approach based solely upon plasma concentration data. Strong emphasis should be placed on both the patient's clinical response and plasma concentration to arrive at an optimal dosage regimen.

⇨ *Single dose pharmacokinetic studies.* Single dose studies involving carbamazepine are of limited value. No consideration for auto-induction is made and the results should be interpreted accordingly.

⇨ *Stress compliance.* A considerable amount of time is spent on gradually increasing the dose to arrive at an optimal regimen. The patient must be made aware of the importance of staying compliant with the regimen. Deviations from this regimen can affect the efficacy of other concomitant medications.

References

1. Winter ME. Basic Clinical Pharmacokinetics. 3rd ed. Vancouver: Applied Therapeutics; 1994:177–184.

2. Levy RH et al. Carbamazepine, Valproic Acid, Phenobarbital, and Ethosuximide. In: Evans WE et al., eds. Applied Pharmacokinetics: Principles of Therapeutic Drug Monitoring. 3rd ed. Vancouver: Applied Therapeutics; 1992: 26-1–26-29.

3. Mikati M. The newer antiepileptic drugs: carbamazepine and valproic acid. Pediatr Ann. 1991;20:34–40.

Notes:

Cyclosporine 3

Cyclosporine is a neutral, hydrophobic cyclic peptide composed of 11 amino acids. It is used to prevent graft-versus-host disease in bone marrow transplant patients and to prevent graft rejection in solid organ transplant patients. Cyclosporine also has been used to delay disease progression in patients with various autoimmune diseases. The impact of cyclosporine in the transplantation arena has been significant. For example, the number of cardiac transplants in the United States increased about 100-fold from 1976 to 1990. Much of this increase can be attributed to cyclosporine. While cyclosporine is relatively non-toxic compared to other immunosuppressants, it does cause significant concentration-related toxicity (primarily nephrotoxicity). Therapeutic concentration monitoring is the standard of practice, since efficacy and toxicity are linked to drug concentrations. Two technical factors which alter the target concentration must be considered in any discussion of cyclosporine plasma concentration monitoring: the biologic fluid measured and the analytical method employed, both of which vary from institution to institution. Target whole blood concentrations generally are 2–3 times greater than plasma concentrations. Target ranges are similar when the monoclonal radioimmunoassay, monoclonal florescence polarization immunoassay, or HPLC are employed; however, the target concentration is 3 times higher when the polyclonal florescence polarization immunoassay is used. Additionally, target concentration ranges differ based upon the institution, the individual practitioner, and the type of transplantation. Lastly, there is a great deal of inter- and intra-individual variability in each of the pharmacokinetic parameters of cyclosporine.

Dose

Initial Dose

⇨ Adults and adolescents.

□ oral: 12–15 mg/kg/day starting 4–12 hr before transplant surgery. Usually, this dose is continued for 1–2 wk postoperatively, at which time the dose slowly is reduced by 5% per week until the maintenance dose is reached

⇨ Adults and adolescents.

□ IV: 2–6 mg/kg/day starting 4–12 hr before surgery and postoperatively until the patient can tolerate oral medication

Maintenance Dose

⇨ Adults and adolescents.

□ oral: 5–10 mg/kg/day (sometimes in 1–2 divided doses)

⇨ *Note:* Pediatric patients may require significantly higher doses because they clear cyclosporine more rapidly than adults.

Therapeutic & Toxic Range

It is important to note that the therapeutic range is variable. Several factors (e.g., assay type, temperature, biologic fluid, time of sampling) must be considered when evaluating cyclosporine levels.

Assay	Serum/Plasma (ng/mL)	Whole Blood (ng/mL)
Monoclonal radioimmunoassay	50–125	150–400
Fluorescence polarization immunoassay: polyclonal	150–400	200–800
Fluorescence polarization immunoassay: monoclonal	50–125	150–400
HPLC	50–125	150–400

Toxic Concentrations. The purpose of therapeutic monitoring is to reduce the likelihood of toxic side effects while at the same time assuring efficacy. The most problematic of cyclosporine's side effects is nephrotoxicity. There are three forms of nephrotoxicity: transient acute renal failure, protracted acute renal failure, and chronic nephropathy. The transient acute form is completely and quickly reversible with the discontinuation of cyclosporine or a reduction in its dose. Protracted acute renal failure results from repeated transient acute renal failure, and recovery is not complete following the discontinuation of cyclosporine. Chronic nephropathy usually is irreversible. Hypertension and gingival hyperplasia also are relatively common side effects of cyclosporine therapy. Additional, less frequent side effects of cyclosporine therapy include: hematologic disorders, gastrointestinal reactions, hepatotoxicity, tremor, headaches, paresthesias, seizures, and hyperglycemia.

Pharmacokinetic Parameters

Bioavailability (F)

⇨ Oral (olive oil solution or soft gelatin capsules): 30%.

□ *Note:* the reported range of bioavailability is great (5%–90%) and varies between and within subjects. 30% represents a reasonable mean value

⇨ IV: 100%.

Volume of Distribution (Vd)

⇨ Vd = 4–5 L/kg.

□ *Note:* the reported range of bioavailability is great and the above value represents an average

Clearance (Cl) & Half-Life (t½)

⇨ Whole blood clearance: 5–10 mL/kg/min in adults.

□ *Note:* the reported range of bioavailability is great and the above value is simply a reasonable average

⇨ Half-life (t½): 6–12 hr.

Useful Pharmacokinetic Equations

To Revise Kd

$$\text{Kd Revised} = \frac{\ln\left(\dfrac{\text{Cpss min} + \dfrac{(S)(F)(\text{Dose})}{Vd}}{\text{Cpss min}}\right)}{\tau} \qquad \text{(Pg 84)}$$

To Solve for Dose Using the Revised Kd

$$\text{Dose} = \frac{(\text{Cpss min})(Vd)(1 - e^{Kd\tau})}{(S)(F)(e^{-Kd\tau})}$$

*To Calculate a New Dose Based Upon
the Current Steady-State Concentration*

$$\text{Desired Dose} = \frac{\text{Cpss desired}}{\text{Cpss current}} \times \text{current dose}$$

(Pg 194)

Serum Sampling Strategies

As a general rule, trough levels are drawn since they are the most reproducible. Because of the great variability in the pharmacokinetics of cyclosporine, daily or every other day concentration monitoring is reasonable during the first few days of therapy. In stable acute care patients, concentrations can be monitored every 3–5 days. In stable ambulatory patients, monthly levels usually are appropriate.

Dialyzability

⇨ Not dialyzable.

Monitoring Parameters

Subjective

⇨ Dental examination.

Objective

⇨ BUN.

⇨ Creatinine.

⇨ Liver function tests (LFTs).

⇨ Cyclosporine plasma concentrations.

⇨ Blood pressure.

Drug Interactions

⇨ *Anticonvulsants* (e.g., carbamazepine, phenobarbital, phenytoin) have been associated with a reduction in cyclosporine concentration.

⇨ *Azole antifungal drugs* (e.g., fluconazole, itraconazole, ketoconazole) have been associated with an increase in cyclosporine concentration.

⇨ *Calcium channel antagonists* (e.g., diltiazem, nicardipine, verapamil) have been associated with an increase in cyclosporine concentration.

⇨ *Cimetidine* has been associated with an increase in cyclosporine concentration.

⇨ *Erythromycin* has been associated with an increase in cyclosporine concentration.

⇨ *Ethanol* has been associated with an increase in cyclosporine concentration.

⇨ *Imipenem-cilastin* has been associated with an increase in cyclosporine concentration.

⇨ *Nafcillin* has been associated with a reduction in cyclosporine concentration.

⇨ *Norfloxacin* has been associated with an increase in cyclosporine concentration.

⇨ *Rifampin* has been associated with a reduction in cyclosporine concentration.

⇨ *Sulfonamides/trimethoprim* has been associated with a reduction in cyclosporine concentration.

⇨ *Steroid hormones* (e.g., methylprednisolone, methyltestosterone, oral contraceptives, danazol) have been associated with an increase in cyclosporine concentration.

Special Considerations for IV Administration

Cyclosporine concentrate for injection should be diluted in glass bottles with either 5% dextrose or normal saline solution at a ratio of 1 mL cyclosporine concentrate (50 mg/mL) per every 20–100 mL diluent. Polyoxyethylated castor oil, the surfactant in cyclosporine concentrate for injection, may leach diethylhexylphthalate (DEHP) from polyvinyl chloride (PVC) bags or IV lines into the IV solution. Also, PVC lines may retain significant amounts of cyclosporine. Use with caution in patients sensitive to polyoxygenated castor oil.

⇨ Stability: appropriately prepared solutions are stable at room temperature for up to 12 hr.

⇨ Administration: should be administered slowly over 2–6 hr.

References

1. Winter ME. Basic Clinical Pharmacokinetics. 3rd ed. Vancouver: Applied Therapeutics; 1994:185–197.

2. Yee G. Cyclosporine. In: Evans WE et al., eds. Applied Pharmacokinetics: Principles of Therapeutic Drug Monitoring. 3rd ed. Vancouver: Applied Therapeutics; 1992:28-1–28-40.

Notes:

Digoxin

Digoxin is a cardiac glycoside that frequently is used to manage patients with congestive heart failure (CHF) and atrial arrhythmias. Digoxin increases both the force and velocity of myocardial contractions (positive inotropic effect), probably by inhibiting the Na^+/K^+ pump in the myocardial tissue. Digoxin also slows the rate of conduction through the myocardium and prolongs the effective refractory period in patients with atrial arrhythmias; particularly atrial fibrillation.

Past experience with digoxin has provided useful information regarding the relationship between plasma concentrations and efficacy, as well as toxicity. Because digoxin has a narrow therapeutic index, therapeutic monitoring and accurate calculation of dosage regimens are important. In addition, several interactions between digoxin and other drugs or various disease states have been characterized and support the need for pharmacokinetic monitoring. Digitalis (Crystodigin) is another cardiac glycoside with pharmacologic and therapeutic properties similar to digoxin; however, it seldom is used.

Dose

Distribution of digoxin into adipose tissue is poor; thus, all dosage calculations should be based upon ideal body weight (IBW). In patients requiring prompt response, a loading dose should be administered to achieve therapeutic concentrations more rapidly. Like other cardiovascular drugs with a high degree of tissue binding, digoxin has two distinct volume compartments which must be considered in the calculation and administration of the digoxin dosage regimen. The following approach is most frequently employed to initiate digoxin loading and maintenance regimens in the adult patient.

Loading Dose

⇨ Calculate the total digoxin loading dose based upon volume of distribution (Vd) and desired plasma concentration.

⇨ Take into account the appropriate bioavailability factor.

⇨ Give no more than 50% of the total loading dose initially.

⇨ Wait ≈6 hr and give the remaining 50% as two separate doses administered 6 hr apart.

☐ if desired effect is seen or toxicity is encountered, the subsequent doses can be withheld

☐ 6-hr dosing intervals allow for distribution into the tissue so that efficacy or toxicity can be assessed

⇨ *General guideline:* 10–15 µg/kg.

Maintenance Dose

⇨ Calculate an appropriate maintenance dose based upon patient's digoxin Cl, desired concentration, and bioavailability.

⇨ Digoxin Cl is altered in patients with CHF.

⇨ *Be sure to use the correct units when calculating maintenance dose.*

⇨ Doses are typically administered as a single daily dose in the a.m.

⇨ After steady state, any dosage change results in a proportional change in plasma concentration.

⇨ Nomograms can be used to determine the daily dose based upon the digoxin eliminated each day.[3]

  □ percent eliminated/day = 0.20 (Cl_{Cr} in mL/min) + 14%. (See Figure 4.1.)

  □ daily digoxin dose = (% eliminated/day × loading dose)

⇨ *General guideline:* 0.125–0.25 mg/day.

Therapeutic & Toxic Range

In contrast to most other drugs, digoxin's therapeutic and adverse effects are strongly correlated with its concentration in tissues rather than in serum. Therefore, plasma concentrations should only be obtained after digoxin has had the opportunity to fully distribute into the tissues (see Serum Sampling Strategies on page 88).

⇨ *Therapeutic range:* 0.5–2.0 ng/mL (μg/L).

  □ atrial fibrillation requires upper end: 1.0–2.0 ng/mL

  □ CHF patients: 0.5–1.5 ng/mL

⇨ *Toxicity* tends to occur >2.0 ng/mL. Most common adverse reactions include:

  □ GI: nausea, vomiting, anorexia

  □ cardiovascular: ventricular arrhythmias (PVC), heart block, bradycardia

  □ central nervous system (CNS): fatigue, weakness, nightmares, hallucinations

  □ visual: greenish-yellow halos around lights

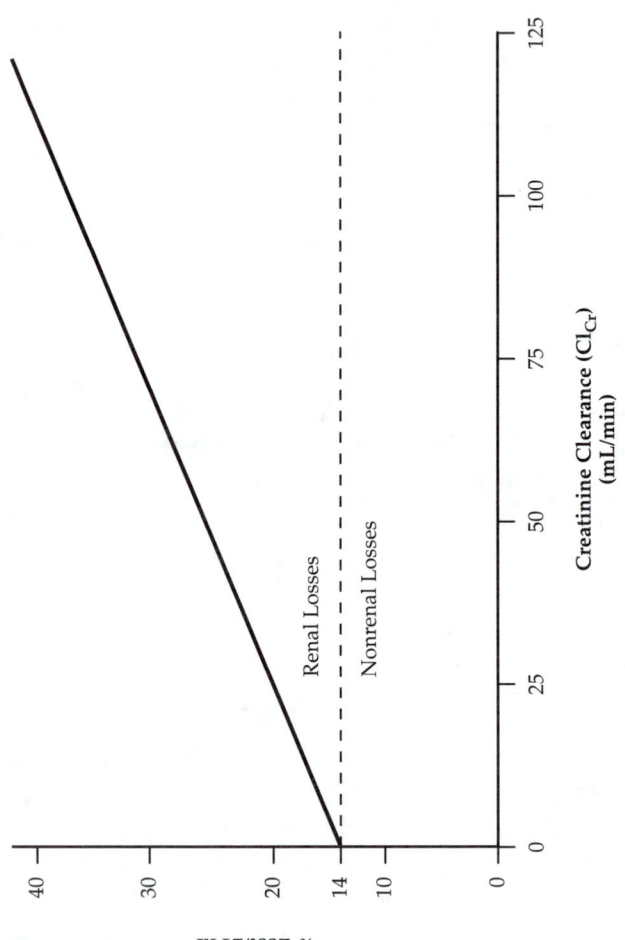

Figure 4.1. Jelliffe method for determining the daily digoxin replacement dose. Reprinted with permission from reference 3.

⇨ Toxicity is greatly enhanced and more severe in the presence of decreased K^+ (<3.0 mEq/L).

Pharmacokinetic Parameters

Bioavailability (F)

⇨ Several dosage formulations are available for digoxin; bioavailability of each differs.

Formulation	Available Strengths	Bioavailability (F) average (range)
Tablets	0.125, 0.25, and 0.50 mg	0.7 (0.5–0.9)[a]
Elixir	0.05 mg/mL (pediatric dosing)	0.8 (0.75–0.85)
Gelatin capsules	0.05, 0.10, and 0.20 mg	0.95 (0.9–1.0)
IV	0.25 mg/mL	1.0

[a]Note variability.

⇨ Not prepared as a salt; S = 1.0 (100%).

⇨ Time to peak tissue concentrations:
  □ oral: 2–6 hr
  □ IV: 1–4 hr

⇨ Peak plasma concentrations occur after 60–90 min but do not correlate with effect or toxicity.

⇨ Onset of action after IV is between 5–30 min versus 30–120 min for oral tablets.

⇨ Duration of action is ≈6 days due to the long t½.

⇨ Majority of absorption occurs in the small intestine; several drugs can interfere with the absorption of digoxin (see Drug Interactions on page 90).

⇨ IM injection should be avoided due to severe local irritation and erratic and incomplete absorption.

Volume of Distribution (Vd)

⇨ Very large Vd due to extensive tissue binding.

⇨ Distributes into two distinct compartments:

   □ Vi = 0.7 L/kg (serum)

   □ Vd = 7.3 L/kg (tissues)

⇨ Tissue distribution takes about 3–4 hr ($t\frac{1}{2}_{\alpha}$ = 35 min).

⇨ Efficacy and toxicity correlate best with tissue rather than plasma concentrations.

   □ heart behaves as if in the tissue compartment (Vd)

   □ different than other cardiovascular drugs (i.e., lidocaine)

   □ see **Basic Clinical Pharmacokinetics**, 3rd edition for more information[1]

⇨ Very little distribution into adipose tissue; therefore, base dose in IBW.

⇨ Only 20% of digoxin is bound to plasma proteins (primarily albumin).

⇨ Several factors can influence Vd of digoxin.

Factor	Vd
Renal impairment	$\downarrow \left[3.8 \text{ L/kg(IBW)} + (\text{Cl}_{Cr} \text{ in mL/min})\right]$
Quinidine	$\downarrow (5.3 \text{ L/kg})$
Hypothyroidism	$\downarrow (3.0 \text{ L/kg})$
Hyperthyroidism	$\uparrow (9.5 \text{ L/kg})$

Clearance (Cl) & Half-Life (t½)

⇨ Digoxin Cl is dependent upon both the kidneys (70%–80%) and the liver (25%); hepatic metabolism may be increased up to 75% in chronic renal failure.

　□ $\text{Cl}_{renal} = \text{Cl}_{Cr}$ as mL/min

　□ $\text{Cl}_{hepatic} = 0.8$ mL/kg/min

　□ $\text{Cl}_{total} = \text{Cl}_{Cr}$ as mL/min $+ (0.8$ mL/kg/min) (weight in kg) *or* 1.02 Cl_{Cr} as mL/min $+ 57$ mL/min (based upon 70 kg)

⇨ Reduction in hepatic blood flow will greatly decrease digoxin Cl in patients with CHF.

　□ Cl_{total} (CHF) $= (0.33$ mL/kg/min)(weight in kg) $+ (0.9) (\text{Cl}_{Cr}$ as mL/min)

⇨ Several drugs can interact with and influence the Cl of digoxin (see Drug Interactions on page 90).

⇨ t½ averages 42 hr (2 days) and is much longer in patients with compromised renal function.

⇨ The long digoxin t½ means steady state is not reached for 8–10 days.

Useful Pharmacokinetic Equations

Loading Dose for either IV or Oral Regimens

$$\text{Loading Dose} = \frac{(Vd)(Cp)}{(S)(F)} \qquad \text{(Eq 11, pg 19)}$$

⇨ Give 50% of the dose initially, then the remaining 50% as two separate doses 6 hr apart if needed.

Maintenance Dose

$$\text{Maintenance Dose} = \frac{(Cl)(Cpss\ ave)(\tau)}{(S)(F)} \qquad \text{(Eq 16, pg 28)}$$

Serum Sampling Strategies

⇨ Routine levels can be obtained to therapeutically monitor digoxin after 8–10 days (steady state).

⇨ Nonsteady-state concentrations can be obtained if efficacy or toxicity are in question and it is not practical to wait until steady state.

⇨ All plasma concentrations *must be obtained after the dose has been fully distributed into the tissues.*

  □ ≈4 hr after an IV dose

  □ ≈6 hr after an oral dose

⇨ Plasma concentrations obtained before distribution will result in significantly elevated digoxin plasma concentrations that are meaningless and run the risk of being misinterpreted (See **Basic Clinical Pharmacokinetics**, 3rd edition for more information).[1]

⇨ Trough plasma concentrations should be drawn to avoid the distribution phase.

⇨ Some drugs can interfere with specific assays causing artificially elevated digoxin plasma concentrations. Check with your laboratory.

⇨ *Reasons to monitor digoxin plasma concentrations:*

 □ to evaluate a recent change in dosage regimen

 □ to evaluate a poor therapeutic response to an appropriate digoxin dose

 □ to confirm suspicions of toxicity

 □ to detect potential drug interactions or bioavailability problems

 □ to assess patient compliance

Dialyzability

Hemodialysis & Peritoneal

⇨ Digoxin plasma concentrations transiently decrease; digoxin is not significantly removed by dialysis.

Hemoperfusion

⇨ Hemoperfusion can remove a small percentage of digoxin from the serum.

Monitoring Parameters

Subjective

⇨ Complaints of side effects (e.g., CNS, visual problems).

⇨ Consider all concurrent medications for drug interactions.

Objective

⇨ Digoxin plasma concentrations.

⇨ Electrocardiogram (ECG): assess therapeutic effect of digoxin; detect the development of new arrhythmias.

⇨ Routine electrolytes (especially K^+).

⇨ BUN/SrCr.

Drug Interactions

⇨ *Quinidine.* The Vd and Cl of digoxin are greatly reduced by quinidine and this results in a two- to three-fold elevation in digoxin plasma concentration. If quinidine is to be added, discontinue the daily digoxin dose for one day and then restart the digoxin at 50% the original dose. Follow plasma concentrations closely.

⇨ *Verapamil, amiodarone, and spironolactone* elevate digoxin plasma concentrations by reducing digoxin Cl. Monitor digoxin plasma concentrations and anticipate a reduction in digoxin dose. Spironolactone may also interfere with digoxin assays.

⇨ *Antacids, cholestyramine, and kaolin-pectin.* Concurrent administration may reduce the extent of digoxin absorption by 30%–60%. Attempt to administer digoxin 1–2 hr before or 2–3 hr after the interacting agents.

⇨ *Please refer to a detailed reference (like* **Drug Interactions & Updates Quarterly**[4]) for other digoxin drug interactions.

Special Considerations

Alternate Day Dosing.   Patients requiring a daily oral dose of digoxin that cannot be easily administered based upon available dosage strengths (i.e., 0.190 mg daily dose) may benefit from alternate day therapy. For example, patients can be instructed to take 0.125 mg QOD (M-W-F-Sun) alternating with 0.25 mg QOD (T-Th-Sat) for an average daily dose of 0.190 mg.

Digoxin Overdose.   In patients who have ingested potentially toxic doses of digoxin, the following steps should be considered:

⇨ Discontinue digoxin.

⇨ Activated charcoal may help to decrease absorption of digoxin.

⇨ Associated arrhythmias should be managed with an appropriate agent (lidocaine).

⇨ Evaluate serum K^+ and administer supplemental K^+ for levels <3.0 mEq/L.

⇨ In life-threatening cases consider administration of digoxin immune Fab (Digibind) IV.

  □ dose of Digibind is based upon estimated amount of digoxin ingested or digoxin plasma concentration

  □ one 40 mg vial of Digibind will bind ≈0.6 mg digoxin

  □ expensive therapy; use only for life-threatening cases

□ calculation based upon amount of digoxin ingested:

$$\text{Dose (mg)} = \frac{(\text{Dose ingested in mg})(F)}{0.6} \times 40$$

□ calculation based upon digoxin plasma concentration:

$$\text{Dose (mg)} = \frac{(\text{Cp as ng/mL})(\text{IBW in kg})}{100} \times 40$$

References

1. Winter ME. Basic Clinical Pharmacokinetics. 3rd ed. Vancouver: Applied Therapeutics; 1994:198–235.

2. Reuning RH et al. Digoxin. In: Evans WE et al, eds. Applied Pharmacokinetics: Principles of Therapeutic Drug Monitoring. 3rd ed. Vancouver: Applied Therapeutics; 1992:20-1–20-48.

3. Jelliffe RW. An improved method of digoxin therapy. Ann Intern Med. 1968;69:703–17.

4. Hansten PD, Horn JR. Drug Interactions & Updates Quarterly. Vancouver: Applied Therapeutics; 1993:495–506.

Notes:

Ethosuximide   5

Ethosuximide is a well-tolerated anticonvulsant used to treat absence seizures exclusively. Additional anticonvulsant agents are required for patients with other types of seizures. Methsuximide and phensuximide also belong to the succinimide class of anticonvulsants; however, their use is limited because they are more toxic and less effective.

Dose

Loading Dose

> ⇨ None required.

Maintenance Dose

> ⇨ General dosage recommendation: 20 mg/kg/day.
>
> ⇨ Therapy is initiated slowly and gradually increased to minimize GI side effects.
>> □ adults: start with 250 mg BID
>> □ children (3–6 yr): start with 250 mg QD
>> □ increase by 250 mg every 4–7 days until desired response is observed
>> □ daily dosage should not exceed 1500 mg without close monitoring
>
> ⇨ After steady state is reached, any change in dose should result in a proportional change in plasma concentration.
>> □ disproportionately higher serum increases have been reported in some patients

⇨ Dosage may require adjustment in patients with impaired hepatic function.

Therapeutic & Toxic Range

⇨ Therapeutic range varies widely: 40–100 mg/L.

⇨ Efficacy correlates well with plasma concentration; concentrations >40 mg/L tend to result in good seizure control in most patients.

⇨ Toxicity is minimal and appears independent of plasma concentrations (except GI complaints); concentrations well above 100 mg/L have not been associated with a higher incidence of toxicity.

⇨ Most common adverse effects include:

   □ GI complaints: nausea, vomiting, diarrhea, abdominal pain

   □ mild central nervous system (CNS): headache, dizziness, confusion, behavior changes

⇨ Rare adverse events: serious blood dyscrasias, systemic lupus erythematosus (SLE), and Stevens-Johnson syndrome.

Pharmacokinetic Parameters

Bioavailability (F)

⇨ Available formulations include:

   □ capsules: 250 mg

   □ solution: 250 mg/5 mL

⇨ Well absorbed with bioavailability approaching 100%.

⇨ Poorly extracted by liver (low extraction ratio); minimal first-pass effect.

⇨ Plasma concentrations peak 2–4 hr after an oral dose.

⇨ Not formulated as a salt (S = 1.0).

Volume of Distribution (Vd)

⇨ Average: Vd = 0.7 L/kg.

⇨ Minimal protein binding allows for rapid and excellent penetration into cerebrospinal fluid (CSF).

⇨ Concentrations in the plasma, CSF, saliva, and breast milk are all similar.

Clearance (Cl) & Half-Life (t½)

⇨ Majority is metabolized by the liver to inactive metabolites.

⇨ 20% is eliminated unchanged in the urine.

⇨ Cl and t½ vary significantly and tend to be age dependent.

Clearance (Cl) and Half-Life (t½)		
	Adults	*Children*
Clearance (Cl)	0.23 L/kg/day	0.39 L/kg/day
Half-life (t½)	50 hr	30 hr

Serum Sampling Strategies

⇨ Optimal regimen should be based primarily upon clinical response as opposed to plasma concentrations.

⇨ No real correlation between toxicity and plasma concentrations.

⇨ Primary reasons for monitoring levels are to:
- ☐ document efficacy
- ☐ evaluate patient compliance
- ☐ assess therapy after the addition or deletion of other anticonvulsant agents

⇨ Steady-state conditions are achieved at 4–7 days in children and up to 10–12 days in adults.

⇨ Timing of sample collection is not critical due to long t½, but should be consistent (e.g., just before dose).

Dialyzability

Hemodialysis

⇨ Ethosuximide is removed by hemodialysis; however, the extent of this elimination has not been fully characterized.

⇨ Reports suggest that ≈50% of ethosuximide is cleared during a 6 hr dialysis.

Monitoring Parameters

Subjective

⇨ Seizure control or seizure frequency.

⇨ Compliance.

Objective

⇨ Ethosuximide plasma concentrations.

⇨ Vital signs.

⇨ White blood cell (WBC) count and differential.

⇨ Platelets.

⇨ Liver function tests (LFTs).

Drug Interactions

⇨ *Valproic acid* can increase ethosuximide plasma concentrations by competitive inhibition of hepatic enzymes.

⇨ *Carbamazepine.* Enhanced metabolism of ethosuximide has been reported.

Special Considerations

⇨ Discontinue therapy gradually to avoid breakthrough seizures.

References

1. Winter ME. Basic Clinical Pharmacokinetics. 3rd ed. Vancouver: Applied Therapeutics; 1994;236–241.

2. Levy RH et al. Carbamazepine, Valproic Acid, Phenobarbital, and Ethosuximide. In: Evans WE et al., eds. Applied Pharmacokinetics: Principles of Therapeutic Drug Monitoring. 3rd ed. Vancouver: Applied Therapeutics; 1992:26-1–26-29.

Lidocaine 6

Lidocaine is classified as a type IB antiarrhythmic agent and is the drug of choice for many serious ventricular arrhythmias. In contrast to other antiarrhythmics, lidocaine's activity is directed solely at the His-Purkinje network with very little effect on the sinoatrial (SA) and atrioventricular (AV) nodes. Lidocaine has little impact on atrial arrhythmias and only is used for arrhythmias involving the ventricles. In addition to its cardiovascular properties, lidocaine is frequently used as an anesthetic agent. The relatively narrow therapeutic index of lidocaine, coupled with several factors that can influence its pharmacokinetic parameters, makes pharmacokinetic monitoring of lidocaine an important consideration.

Tocainide and mexiletine are oral antiarrhythmic agents that share the IB classification with lidocaine; however, these agents are not as valuable for managing acute situations and are reserved for chronic therapy.

Dose

Loading Dose

Due to lidocaine's unique two-compartment distribution characteristics, special consideration is required when calculating dosage regimens. Because the efficacy and toxicity of lidocaine correlates with plasma rather than tissue concentrations, the initial loading dose must be based on the initial volume of distribution (Vi). If volume of distribution (Vd) is used, the initial concentration of lidocaine obtained in the plasma will exceed the upper limit of the therapeutic range and greatly increase the potential for toxicity. (See Figures 6.1 and 6.2.)

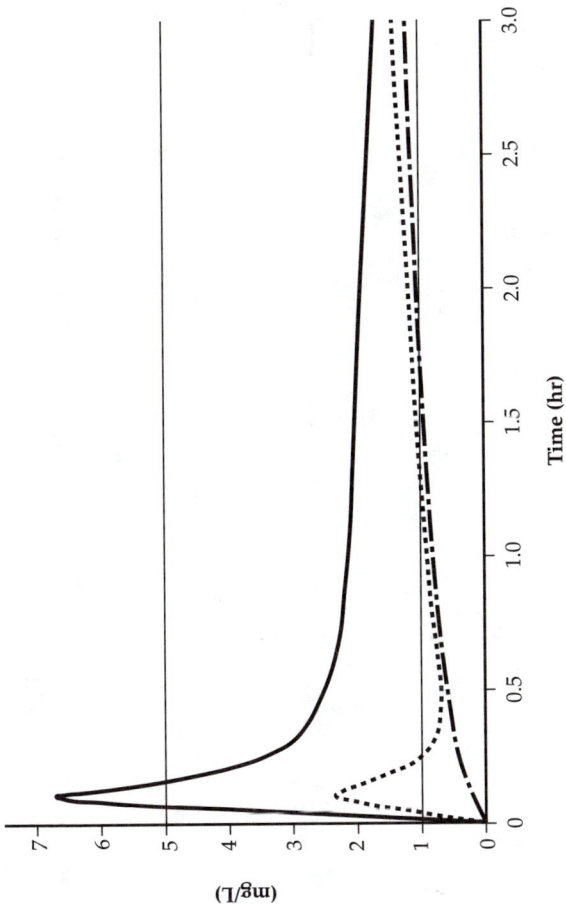

Figure 6.1. Lidocaine plasma concentrations associated with three different dosage regimens: (—) loading dose based upon Vd plus an infusion; (- - -) loading dose based upon Vi plus an infusion; (– –) infusion only with no loading dose.

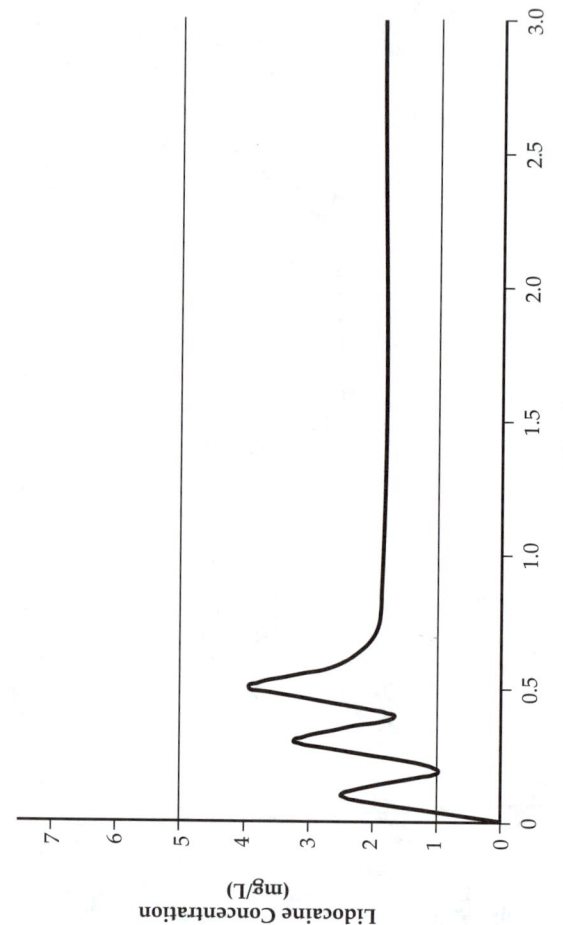

Figure 6.2. Lidocaine plasma concentrations associated with the use of "mini-boluses" in addition to a constant infusion.

⇨ Loading dose = 1–2 mg/kg, based upon ideal body weight (IBW); repeat as needed.

⇨ The initial loading dose will quickly distribute into the tissues.

⇨ Subsequent "mini-boluses" usually are employed to maintain concentrations in the therapeutic range until the maintenance infusion produces the desired plasma concentration. (See Figure 6.2.)

⇨ "Mini-boluses" should be repeated every 15 min until:

   □ the desired response is achieved or toxicity is encountered

   □ the total loading dose (based upon Vd) has been administered

Maintenance Dose

⇨ Maintenance dose = 1–4 mg/min via continuous IV infusion.

⇨ Usual IM dose = 300 mg (or 4.3 mg/kg).

Therapeutic & Toxic Range

Therapeutic and toxic effects of lidocaine are closely correlated with concentrations achieved in the plasma. Unlike the aminoglycosides or digoxin, acute changes in plasma concentrations will result in acute changes in either efficacy or toxicity of lidocaine.

⇨ *Therapeutic range:* 1–5 mg/L.

⇨ Mild central nervous system (CNS) effects (e.g., confusion, dizziness, visual disturbances): >5 mg/L, but may occur as low as 3–5 mg/L.

⇨ **Serious toxicity** (e.g., cardiovascular depression, tremors, seizures, coma): >8–9 mg/L.

⇨ Elderly and patients with recent acute myocardial infarction (MI) or congestive heart failure (CHF) are at higher risk for lidocaine toxicity.

⇨ The contribution of active lidocaine metabolites to toxicity is unclear.

Pharmacokinetic Parameters

Bioavailability (F)

⇨ Oral absorption is rapid, but extensive first-pass metabolism limits its utility.

⇨ Lidocaine is administered by IV or IM to avoid first-pass metabolism.

　□ immediate onset of action with IV route; duration of action is ≈15–20 min

　□ rapid onset with IV is useful in acute settings

　□ peak concentrations take longer following IM injections; Cpss max is higher in deltoid versus gluteal injections

⇨ Rectal administration (F = 0.7) also can be utilized to overcome first-pass effect.

⇨ Systemic absorption is possible when used as a local anesthetic.

⇨ Salt fraction (S) = 1.0.

Volume of Distribution (Vd)

⇨ Widely distributed and extensively bound to tissues and proteins.

⇨ Protein binding is 60%–80% (⅔ to α-1-acid glycoprotein; ⅓ to albumin).

⇨ Factors that affect protein binding can alter lidocaine volume. (See **Basic Clinical Pharmacokinetics**, 3rd edition for more information.)[1]

⇨ Initially distributed into plasma or initial compartment (V_i = 0.5 L/kg).

⇨ Volume greatly expands as lidocaine is distributed into tissues or tissue compartment (V_d = 1.3 L/kg).

⇨ Plasma concentration will drop substantially as lidocaine distributes into tissues; therefore, additional "mini-boluses" are required.

⇨ *Factors that can influence lidocaine V_d:*

	V_i (L/kg)	V_d (L/kg)
Normal	0.5	1.3
CHF	↓ 0.3	↓ 0.88
Cirrhosis	↑ 0.61	↑ 2.3

Clearance (Cl) & Half-Life (t½)

⇨ >90% metabolized by the liver.

⇨ Highly extracted drug (extraction ratio >0.7); clearance (Cl) is primarily flow dependent.

⇨ Two main metabolites monoethylglycine xylidide (MEGX) (80%–90% active) and glycine xylidide (GX) (10%–20% active).

⇨ Lidocaine Cl = 10 mL/min/kg.

⇨ *Factors that influence lidocaine Cl:*

	$t\frac{1}{2}$ (hr)	Lidocaine Cl (mL/min/kg)
Normal	1.5–2	10
CHF	1.5–2	↓6
Cirrhosis	5	↓6
Acute MI	4	9

⇨ Impaired renal function has little effect upon lidocaine Cl and $t\frac{1}{2}$.

⇨ Distribution phase ($t\frac{1}{2}\alpha$) = 10 min.

   □ initial dose is completely distributed after 3–5 $t\frac{1}{2}\alpha$ (30–60 min)

⇨ Elimination $t\frac{1}{2}$ = 1.5–2 hr.

   □ $t\frac{1}{2}$ may become prolonged when continuous infusions run beyond 24–48 hr

Useful Pharmacokinetic Equations

⇨ Cirrhosis and CHF may influence Vd and Cl values for lidocaine.

Initial Loading Dose

$$\text{Initial Loading Dose} = \frac{(Vi)(Cpss\ max\ desired)}{(S)(F)}$$

Total Loading Dose

$$\text{Total Loading Dose} = \frac{(Vd)(Cpss\ max\ desired)}{(S)(F)}$$

Maintenance Infusion

$$\text{Rate of Maintenance Dose} = \frac{(Cl)(Cpss\ ave\ desired)}{(S)(F)}$$

Serum Sampling Strategies

⇨ Lidocaine is used in acute settings where efficacy usually can be assessed based upon clinical response [i.e., electrocardiogram (ECG)].

⇨ Serum levels are more useful as a gauge for toxicity, rather than efficacy.

⇨ When necessary, samples should be obtained after steady state is reached ($\approx$10 hr).

⇨ Plasma concentrations are particularly useful in:

  □ patients with reduced or changing Cl

  □ unconscious patients in which CNS toxicity may not be easily assessed

  □ patients who are therapeutically unresponsive despite maximal lidocaine doses

⇨ *In vitro* interactions can occur when serum samples are collected in tubes containing the plasticizer TBEP; however, most currently available collection tubes have replaced TBEP with an inert material.

Dialyzability

Hemodialysis & Peritoneal

> ⇨ The influence of hemodialysis and peritoneal dialysis on lidocaine remains unclear.

> ⇨ Due to the short duration of action and its use in the acute setting, the clinical impact of dialysis is minimal.

Monitoring Parameters

Subjective

> ⇨ Increased agitation.

> ⇨ Complaints of dizziness, confusion.

> ⇨ Tremors, seizures.

Objective

> ⇨ ECG monitoring.

> ⇨ Vital signs.

> ⇨ Serum electrolytes.

> ⇨ Lidocaine plasma concentrations.

> ⇨ Altered mentation.

Drug Interactions

> ⇨ *Other cardiovascular agents.* Lidocaine can potentiate the cardiac depressive effects of other cardiovascular agents when administered concomitantly.

⇨ *Propranolol and metoprolol.* β-blockade reduction in cardiac output can reduce systemic Cl of lidocaine by 30%–50%.

⇨ *Cimetidine.* 20%–25% reduction in lidocaine Cl with co-administration of cimetidine may occur. A similar reduction was not seen with ranitidine.

⇨ *Protein binding.* Drugs such as anticonvulsants, quinidine, and oral contraceptives can influence the protein binding of lidocaine.

Special Considerations

⇨ IV infusions of lidocaine should be administered at a rate not to exceed 50 mg/min.

⇨ Lidocaine preparations containing epinephrine (commonly used for anesthetic purposes) should *NOT* be administered intravenously for treating arrhythmias.

⇨ Lidocaine is compatible with most IV fluids (see more detailed references for specific compatibility information).

References

1. Winter ME. Basic Clinical Pharmacokinetics. 3rd ed. Vancouver: Applied Therapeutics; 1994:242–256.

2. Pieper JA, Johnson KE. Lidocaine. In: Evans WE et al., eds. Applied Pharmacokinetics: Principles of Therapeutic Drug Monitoring. 3rd ed. Vancouver: Applied Therapeutics; 1992: 21-1–21-35.

Lithium   7

Lithium salts are used to treat bipolar affective disorder and acute mania. They also have been used to treat inappropriate secretion of antidiuretic hormone. Several theoretical mechanisms of action have been proposed, including lithium's interference with similar ions such as sodium, potassium, magnesium, and calcium to produce membrane stabilization and inhibit intracellular messengers.

The therapeutic window of lithium is small (i.e., 0.8–1.5 mEq/L). Concentrations >1.5 mEq/L are associated with central nervous system (CNS) side effects such as lethargy, muscle weakness, fatigue, and tremor. Therapeutic monitoring of this medication is essential since several dynamic factors, including sodium loading or depletion and renal function, influence the elimination of this compound.

Dose

⇨ Adults: 900–1200 mg/day in 2–3 divided doses.

Therapeutic & Toxic Range

Therapeutic Range

⇨ Acute mania: 1.0–1.5 mEq/L.

⇨ Chronic therapy: 0.8–1.2 mEq/L.

Toxic Plasma Concentrations: >1.5 mEq/L

Toxic Symptoms:

⇨ **CNS.** Lethargy, weakness, tremor, and confusion are suggestive of toxic concentrations.

⇨ *Cardiac.* T wave changes are quite common (e.g., 20%–30%) but usually are not problematic. Arrhythmias may be observed, but are rare.

⇨ *GI.* Nausea, vomiting, diarrhea, and abdominal pain. An extended-release product may decrease the severity of nausea and vomiting. Diarrhea may be less severe if patients are treated with a rapidly-absorbed dosage form.

⇨ Metallic taste.

⇨ Polydipsia/Polyuria.

⇨ Hyperthyroidism.

⇨ Weight gain.

Pharmacokinetic Parameters

Bioavailability (F)

⇨ Oral products are completely absorbed (F = 1.0).

Lithium Products

Formulation	Available Strengths	
Lithium carbonate tablets	300 mg	8.12 mEq
Lithium carbonate capsules	150 mg	4.06 mEq
Lithium carbonate capsules	300 mg	8.12 mEq
Lithium carbonate capsules	600 mg	16.24 mEq
Lithium carbonate tablets (slow release)	300 mg	8.12 mEq
Lithium carbonate tablets (controlled release)	450 mg	12.18 mEq
Lithium citrate syrup	—	8 mEq/5 cc

⇨ *Time to peak concentrations:*

  □ capsules and tablets: 1–2 hr

  □ sustained-release tablets: 4–5 hr

⇨ Salt fraction (S) = 1.0 (mEq amounts used in equations).

Volume of Distribution (Vd)

⇨ Lithium distribution may be described by a two-compartment model with the alpha volume of distribution ranging from 0.25–0.3 L/kg. Concentrations measured during the alpha phase do not correlate with toxicity or with efficacy.

⇨ The average final Vd = 0.7 L/kg.

Clearance (Cl) & Half-Life (t½)

⇨ Lithium is filtered by the glomerulus and reabsorbed in the renal tubules like other divalent cations; important for drug and food interactions.

⇨ Cl = $(0.25)(Cl_{Cr})$.

⇨ *Factors that increase Cl:*

  □ pregnancy

  □ sodium supplements

⇨ *Factors that decrease Cl:*

  □ renal dysfunction

  □ dehydration

□ hyponatremia: patients should not be sodium restricted and should try to maintain a consistent intake of sodium

⇨ $\alpha t\frac{1}{2} \approx 6$ hr.

⇨ $\beta t\frac{1}{2} \approx 20$ hr.

Useful Pharmacokinetic Equations

Steady-State Concentrations

$$\text{Cpss ave} = \frac{(S)(F)(\text{Dose}/\tau)}{Cl} \qquad \text{(Eq 35, pg 46)}$$

mEq to mg Conversion

$$\frac{\text{Lithium Dose}}{(\text{mEq})} = \left(\begin{array}{c}\text{Lithium Carbonate Dose}\\(\text{mg})\end{array}\right)\left(\frac{8.12\ \text{mEq}}{300\ \text{mg}}\right)$$
$$\text{(Eq 7.2, pg 261)}$$

Serum Sampling Strategies

⇨ Samples should be obtained just before a dose (at least 12 hr after the last dose).

⇨ Additional samples (at a later date) should be taken at the same time during the day.

⇨ The $\beta t\frac{1}{2}$ in most patients is ≈ 18 hr; thus, steady state will be reached in 3–5 days.

⇨ Some clinicians suggest pharmacokinetic evaluations after the first dose.

⇨ Therapeutic effect may not be apparent for 2–3 weeks.

⇨ *Other indications for plasma concentrations:*

   □ to assess possible toxicity

   □ after dose changes

   □ altered renal function

   □ electrolyte imbalances

   □ weekly during pregnancy

   □ in the event of a psychiatric relapse

Dialyzability

Hemodialysis

⇨ Significant removal.

Peritoneal

⇨ Significant removal.

Monitoring Parameters

Subjective

⇨ Signs and symptoms of bipolar affective disorder.

⇨ Lethargy/fatigue.

⇨ Nausea/vomiting.

⇨ Metallic taste.

Objective

⇨ Renal function tests.

⇨ Electrocardiogram (ECG).

⇨ Serum electrolytes.

⇨ Thyroid function tests.

⇨ Complete blood count (CBC).

⇨ Urinalysis.

⇨ Pregnancy test.

⇨ Tremor.

Drug Interactions

⇨ *Acetazolamide* may increase lithium Cl.

⇨ *Aminophylline* may increase lithium Cl.

⇨ *Caffeine* may increase lithium Cl.

⇨ *Ibuprofen* may decrease lithium Cl.

⇨ *Indomethacin* may decrease lithium Cl.

⇨ *Naproxen* may decrease lithium Cl.

⇨ *Osmotic diuretics* may increase lithium Cl.

⇨ *Sodium supplements* may increase lithium Cl.

⇨ *Theophylline* may increase lithium Cl.

⇨ *Thiazide diuretics* may decrease lithium Cl.

References

1. Winter ME. Basic Clinical Pharmacokinetics. 3rd ed. Vancouver: Applied Therapeutics; 1994:257–265.

2. Amdisen A, Carson SW. Lithium. In: Evans WE et al., eds. Applied Pharmacokinetics: Principles of Therapeutic Drug Monitoring. 3rd ed. Vancouver: Applied Therapeutics; 1992: 34-1–34-26.

Notes:

Methotrexate (MTX)   8

Methotrexate (MTX) is used to treat various forms of leukemia, Wilm's tumor, non-Hodgkin's lymphoma, osteogenic sarcoma, and some autoimmune conditions such as rheumatoid arthritis. MTX is an analog of aminopterin which acts as an antagonist for folic acid (FA) by inhibiting the enzyme, dihydrofolate reductase (DHFR). The enzyme catalyzes the conversion of FA to the reduced or active folate cofactors. Depletion of folate cofactors results in a reduction of DNA synthesis, thus halting cell replication. The complex pharmacokinetics of MTX and the extensive inter-patient variability that exists, coupled with the correlation between MTX concentrations and therapeutic and toxic effects, makes pharmacokinetic monitoring an imperative consideration. MTX levels are primarily monitored in patients receiving high doses used for chemotherapy (i.e., >100 mg/m^2). Patients receiving lower doses generally do not require MTX levels *unless* they have renal failure.

Dose

⇨ Range: 20–12,000 mg.

□ *note:* doses and infusion rates used for cancer therapy vary with protocols and cancer types

□ sarcomas: 12 gm/m^2 over 4 hr

□ leukemia: 40–80 mg/m^2/hr × 24–36°

Therapeutic & Toxic Range

Therapeutic Range

⇨ The majority of regimens target a concentration $>10^{-7}$ molar for <48 hr.

⇨ The therapeutic range varies from 10^{-2} molar to 10^{-6} molar depending upon the condition being treated.

Toxic Concentrations

⇨ Toxicity is observed with plasma concentrations $>1 \times 10^{-8}$ to 1×10^{-7} that persist for longer than 48 hr without the addition of leucovorin rescue.

Signs of Toxicity

⇨ Bone marrow suppression.

⇨ Oral and GI mucositis.

⇨ Hepatic dysfunction.

⇨ Renal dysfunction (not concentration dependent, but *administration* dependent); can be minimized with proper hydration and alkalinization techniques.

⇨ Rash (idiosyncratic, not dose related).

Leucovorin Rescue:

⇨ 10–50 mg/m² Q 6 hr for 12–72 hr or until the MTX concentration $<1 \times 10^{-7}$ molar.

⇨ Doses of <20 mg/m² may be given orally, larger doses should be administered by IV because of capacity-limited absorption.

⇨ In cases where MTX concentrations exceed 1×10^{-6} at 48 hr, leucovorin dose should be increased to 50–100 mg/m² and the interval reduced to 4 hr to minimize MTX toxicity.

Pharmacokinetic Parameters

Bioavailability (F)

⇨ Absorption is capacity limited:

☐ doses <30 mg/m²: F = 1.0

☐ doses >80 mg/m²: F is variable; IV administration recommended

⇨ Time to peak concentrations: 1–2 hr after low oral dose.

⇨ Commercial MTX is not a salt (S = 1.0).

Volume of Distribution (Vd)

⇨ Vi = 0.2–0.5 L/kg.

⇨ Vd = 0.7 L/kg.

⇨ The presence of ascites, edema, or pleural effusions will increase Vd but, more significantly, will increase the terminal beta half-life ($\beta t\frac{1}{2}$).

Clearance (Cl) & Half-Life (t½)

⇨ MTX is cleared for the most part by a renal mechanism; it is both filtered and secreted by the renal tubules, an important factor in drug interactions.

☐ MTX Cl = (1.6)(Cl_{Cr}).

⇨ Hepatic metabolism does occur but is relatively insignificant and thus, is not included in the estimation of total clearance.

□ one hepatic metabolite, 7-OH-methotrexate may be an important nephrotoxin

□ alkalinization of the urine with sodium bicarbonate and/or acetazolamide will reduce nephrotoxicity by increasing elimination of the metabolite

⇨ t½ varies because Vd and Cl change with concentration:

□ for concentrations $>5 \times 10^{-7}$ molar, t½ ≈3 hr

□ for concentrations $<5 \times 10^{-7}$ molar, t½ ≈10 hr

⇨ t½ changes at $\approx 10^{-6}$ molar.

Useful Pharmacokinetic Equations

Conversion of Units

$$\begin{array}{c} \text{MTX Concentration} \\ \text{in mg/L} \end{array} = \left(\begin{array}{c} \text{MTX Concentration} \\ \text{in } 10^{-6} \text{ Molar} \end{array}\right)(0.454)$$

(Eq 8.2, pg 268)

Equivalent Units

⇨ 0.01×10^{-4} molar.

⇨ 0.1×10^{-5} molar.

⇨ 1.0×10^{-6} molar.

⇨ 1 micro molar.

⇨ 10×10^{-7} molar.

⇨ 0.454 mg/L.

Continuous Infusion (See **Basic Clinical Pharmacokinetics,** *3rd edition pp. 274–279 for more information.*[1])

24-hour concentration

Note: This equation is useful *only* if MTX is given as a continuous infusion. If given as a bolus, must use bolus-dose equation; then, which Vd to use becomes controversial. The second equation combines the two equations found on page 276 of **Basic Clinical Pharmacokinetics**, 3rd edition.

$$\text{Cpss ave in mg/L} = \frac{(S)(F)(Dose/\tau)}{Cl} \qquad \text{(Eq 35, pg 46)}$$

or

$$\text{Cpss ave in } 10^{-6} \text{ Molar} = \frac{\dfrac{(S)(F)(Dose/\tau)}{Cl}}{0.454} \qquad \text{(Pg 276)}$$

48-hour concentration

$$Cp = \text{Cpss ave } (e^{-Kdt})$$

where: t = the time interval spanning from the end of the infusion to the 48-hr sampling time

This equation is used to predict the concentration 48 hr after the beginning of the 36 hr infusion where Cpss ave is the concentration at the end of the infusion and t is 12 hr (48 hr – 36 hr). The Kd value may be estimated by use of the equation: $Kd = 0.693/t\frac{1}{2} = 0.231 \text{ hr}^{-1}$, assuming a 3 hr $t\frac{1}{2}$ during this first period of two-compartment elimination. The 3 hr $t\frac{1}{2}$ should be used until a concentration of 0.5×10^{-7} molar is reached.

60-hr concentration

$$Cp = Cp^0(e^{-Kdt}) \qquad \text{(Eq 26, pg 37)}$$

This equation is used to predict the concentration 60 hr after the beginning of the 36 hr infusion, where Cp is the concentration at 48 hr and t is 12 hr (48 hr – 36 hr). The Kd value may be estimated by use of the equation: $Kd = 0.693/t\frac{1}{2} = 0.231\ hr^{-1} = 0.0693\ hr^{-1}$, assuming a 10 hr t½ during this second period of the two-compartment elimination. The 10 hr t½ may be used after the concentration drops below 0.5×10^{-7}.

The following equation may be used to predict the time required for the MTX concentration to drop below 1.0×10^{-7}.

$$t = \frac{\ln\left(\dfrac{Cp_1}{Cp_2}\right)}{Kd} \qquad \text{(Eq 4.6, pg 215)}$$

⇨ The Kd value used in the above equation should be derived from the decay from 48–60 hr.

Serum Sampling Strategies

Sampling times vary depending upon the protocol; however, one should obtain a concentration after steady state has been achieved during the infusion, at 48 hr, and every 24 hr thereafter until rescue is complete.

Dialyzability

Hemodialysis

⇨ Conventional: 30–40 mL/min.

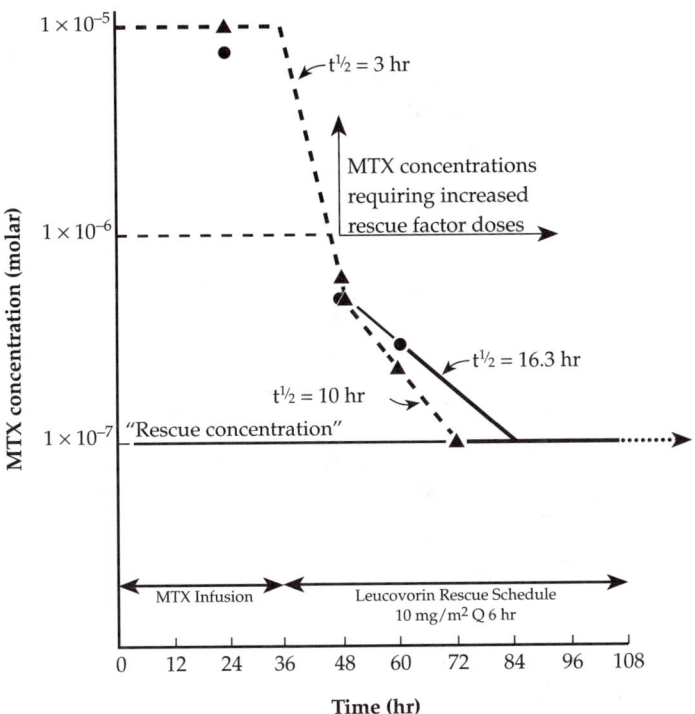

Figure 8.1. Methotrexate. This figure represents a semilog plot of the expected (▲) and measured (●) methotrexate (MTX) plasma concentrations during and following a 36 hr infusion. Levels were obtained at 24, 48, and 60 hr after the start of the infusion. Note that leucovorin rescue should be continued as long as the MTX concentration is greater than the rescue value (represented here as 1×10^{-7} molar or 0.1 micromolar) and that the rescue dose should be increased for MTX levels greater than 1×10^{-6} molar at 48 hr and beyond.

Monitoring Parameters

Subjective

⇨ Nausea/vomiting (usually mild to moderate): may be controlled with antiemetics.

Objective

⇨ Plasma concentrations.

⇨ Renal function.

  □ urine output

  □ urine pH

  □ renal function tests (e.g., BUN, Cl_{Cr})

  □ hematuria

⇨ Myelosuppression.

  □ leukopenia

  □ thrombocytopenia

  □ anemia

  □ nadir usually occurs 7–10 days post dose

⇨ Liver function tests (LFTs).

⇨ Rash.

Drug Interactions

⇨ *Antibiotics (oral)* may decrease the absorption of MTX resulting in reduced plasma concentrations.

⇨ *Aspirin* may reduce the Cl and the protein binding of MTX.

⇨ *Diclofenac.* Concurrent therapy with MTX may increase the toxicity of MTX in patients with renal dysfunction.

⇨ *NSAIDs.* These drugs may reduce the Cl of MTX in some patients resulting in prolonged exposure to high concentrations.

⇨ *Probenecid* may reduce the renal clearance (Cl_r) of MTX.

⇨ *Sulfonamides* may reduce the Cl_r of MTX.

Special Considerations for IV Administration

⇨ Lyophilized MTX should be reconstituted with preservative-free normal saline (PFNS).

⇨ MTX for intrathecal administration should *always* be reconstituted with PFNS or Elliott's B solution.

⇨ A sodium salt form of MTX is available from the National Cancer Institute which may be reconstituted with D5W, NS, or Elliott's B solution.

References

1. Winter ME. Basic Clinical Pharmacokinetics. 3rd ed. Vancouver: Applied Therapeutics; 1994:266–288.

2. Evans WE et al. Methotrexate. In: Evans WE et al., eds. Applied Pharmacokinetics: Principles of Therapeutic Drug Monitoring. 3rd ed. Vancouver: Applied Therapeutics; 1992:29-1–29-42.

3. Hande KR et al. Methotrexate and hemodialysis. Ann Intern Med. 1977;87:495–496.

Phenobarbital   9

Phenobarbital has been used to treat generalized tonic-clonic seizures and partial seizures and to prevent febrile seizures in children. Phenobarbital's unique pharmacokinetic characteristics, the
well-established relationship between its Cp and efficacy and toxicity, and its potential for influencing the disposition of several
other drugs, make therapeutic drug monitoring an important tool.

Dose

The time required to reach steady-state conditions with a maintenance regimen of phenobarbital is about 3–4 weeks because of
its long half-life (t½).

Loading Dose

⇨ An oral or IV loading dose is recommended to achieve
   therapeutic concentrations more rapidly.

   □ base loading dose upon volume of distribution
      (Vd) and desired concentration

   □ give in divided doses to avoid large single dose;
      many clinicians are reluctant to administer ≈1000
      mg as a single dose

   □ give IV load in 3 divided doses at 15–20 min in-
      tervals

   □ the infusion rate should not exceed 50 mg/min

⇨ *General dosing guidelines:* 10–15 mg/kg.

Maintenance Dose

⇨ The maintenance dose should be based upon clearance (Cl) and desired concentration.

⇨ Start with 25% of the full maintenance dose and gradually titrate upward until adequate seizure control is achieved.

⇨ *Common titration schedules are as follows:*

% of Full Maintenance Dose	τ	Duration
25%	Daily	1–2 weeks
↑ to 50%	Daily	1–2 weeks
↑ to 75%	Daily	1–2 weeks
↑ to 100%	Daily	

⇨ Give drug at bedtime to minimize daytime sedation.

⇨ After stabilized on a specific regimen, any dosage change should result in a proportional change in the plasma concentration (unlike carbamazepine).

⇨ *General dosing guidelines:*
  □ adults: 1–3 mg/kg/day
  □ children: 2–5 mg/kg/day

Therapeutic & Toxic Range

Therapeutic Range:

⇨ 10–30 mg/L.

Toxic Levels

⇨ Concentrations exceeding the therapeutic range are associated with toxicity, especially sedation.

⇨ Some patients tolerate high levels with no apparent adverse effects.

⇨ Concentrations >100 mg/L may be fatal.

⇨ Toxicity can be minimized by gradually increasing the dose over time.

⇨ *Primary side effects include:*

   □ sedation (tolerance occurs over time)

   □ ataxia

   □ nystagmus

   □ depression

   □ respiratory depression (overdose)

   □ dermatologic problems

   □ hyperactivity in children

   □ learning difficulties in children

Pharmacokinetic Parameters

Bioavailability (F)

⇨ Available routes of administration include: oral, IV, IM, and rectal.

   □ parenteral product is in the form of sodium phenobarbital (S = 0.91)

   □ several strengths of oral tablets are available ranging from 8–100 mg

   □ elixirs are supplied in 15 mg/5 mL or 20 mg/ 5 mL concentrations

⇨ Oral absorption is fairly complete (F = 0.8–1.0).

⇨ Peak plasma concentrations occur ≈0.5–4 hr after oral doses.

⇨ Rectal administration of phenobarbital may also be utilized (F = 80%).

Volume of Distribution (Vd)

⇨ Average Vd: 0.7 L/kg.

⇨ Distribution into cerebrospinal fluid (CSF) is much slower than other well-perfused organs.

  □ CSF:plasma ratio = 0.50 (correlates with the fraction unbound)

  □ peak CSF concentrations occur after ≈10 hr

  □ not useful in the acute management of status epilepticus

⇨ Protein binding is <50%; phenobarbital is not significantly influenced by other displacing drugs.

Clearance (Cl) & Half-Life (t½)

⇨ 45%–75% is metabolized by the liver to an inactive metabolite.

⇨ 20%–25% is excreted unchanged in the urine.

  □ urine alkalinization and forced diuresis will enhance renal clearance (Cl_r)

⇨ Cl is very slow: 4 mL/kg/hr or 0.1 L/kg/day.

  □ children typically have a faster rate of Cl (up to twofold greater)

  □ activated charcoal is effective in enhancing the Cl of phenobarbital

⇨ Potent inducer of hepatic enzymes.

◻ increases Cl of other hepatically eliminated drugs (see Drug Interactions on page 130)

◻ auto-induction does not appear to occur

◻ Cl is not significantly influenced by other enzyme inducers (except valproic acid)

⇨ t½ averages ≈4–5 days.

⇨ Steady state is not reached until after roughly 2–3 weeks.

Useful Pharmacokinetic Equations

Loading Dose

$$\text{Loading Dose} = \frac{(Vd)(Cp)}{(S)(F)}$$

(Eq 11, pg 19)

Maintenance Dose

$$\text{Maintenance Dose} = \frac{(Cl)(Cpss\ ave)(\tau)}{(S)(F)}$$

(Eq 16, pg 28)

Determination of Nonsteady-State Plasma Concentrations

$$Cp_1 = \frac{(S)(F)(Dose/\tau)}{Cl}(1 - e^{-Kdt_1})$$

(Eq 37, pg 48)

Where: t_1 = The number of hours or days the dose has been given (units must correspond with elimination rate constant). The continuous infusion model can be used because phenobarbital has a long $t\frac{1}{2}$ and narrow peak and trough variations.

Serum Sampling Strategies

⇨ Routine plasma concentrations should only be obtained after steady-state conditions are reached (3–4 weeks).

⇨ If toxicity occurs or seizure activity is not adequately controlled, nonsteady-state levels can be obtained.

⇨ The average steady-state concentration can be estimated by multiplying the phenobarbital dose in mg/kg by 10 (e.g., a 2 mg/kg dose should produce a Cpss ≈20 mg/L).

⇨ Actual sampling time is not critical due to narrow peak and trough variations; however, it is best to be consistent.

⇨ Plasma concentrations should be obtained whenever other anticonvulsants are added or discontinued.

Dialyzability

Hemodialysis & Peritoneal

⇨ Removed by hemodialysis and, to a lesser extent, peritoneal dialysis.

⇨ Dialysis in conjunction with activated charcoal and forced diuresis can be used to manage acute toxicity secondary to overdose.

Hemoperfusion

⇨ Successfully removes phenobarbital.

Monitoring Parameters

Subjective

⇨ Decreased mentation.

⇨ Seizure control or seizure frequency.

⇨ Compliance.

Objective

⇨ Phenobarbital plasma concentrations.

⇨ Vital signs.

⇨ White blood cell (WBC) count.

⇨ Platelets.

⇨ Electroencephalogram (EEG).

Drug Interactions

⇨ Phenobarbital's ability to induce hepatic enzymes results in several drug interactions:

Drugs that ↓ Phenobarbital Cl	Phenobarbital will ↑ Cl of
Valproic acid	Warfarin[a]
Propoxyphene	Phenytoin[b]
	Digoxin
	Corticosteroids
	Oral contraceptives

[a] Abrupt discontinuation of phenobarbital may result in an ↑ risk of hemorrhaging.

[b] Phenobarbital may also ↓ Cl of phenytoin through metabolic inhibition.

Special Considerations

⇨ Phenobarbital infusions should not exceed a rate of 50 mg/min. This avoids the hypotensive effects of the propylene glycol diluent.

⇨ Extravasation of IV sodium phenobarbital can result in significant necrosis of tissue.

⇨ IV sodium phenobarbital is compatible with most non-acid IV fluids; however, several physical and chemical incompatibilities exist and specialized references should be consulted for specific drug incompatibilities.

References

1. Winter ME. Basic Clinical Pharmacokinetics. 3rd ed. Vancouver: Applied Therapeutics; 1994:289–311.

2. Levy RH et al. Carbamazepine, Valproic Acid, Phenobarbital, and Ethosuximide. In: Evans WE et al., eds. Applied Pharmacokinetics: Principles of Therapeutic Drug Monitoring. 3rd ed. Vancouver: Applied Therapeutics; 1992:26-1–26-29.

Notes:

Phenytoin   10

Phenytoin, a hydantoin antiepileptic drug, is effective in treating a broad range of seizures with the exception of absence seizures. It occasionally is used to treat cardiac arrhythmias and diabetic nephropathy. When a rapid effect is required, the concurrent use of lorazepam with a phenytoin loading dose is recommended. Patients may be loaded with oral or IV-administered phenytoin. Peak concentrations and therapeutic effect may not be observed for hours after oral loading doses. A therapeutic lag time of 15–20 minutes usually accompanies IV loading doses as well.

Phenytoin is unique compared to most other medications in that it follows Michaelis-Menten pharmacokinetics and undergoes metabolic degradation via saturable enzyme pathways. Metabolic pathways can become saturated at concentrations that are encountered clinically; therefore, the relationship between dose and plasma concentration is not linear. In addition, the protein binding of phenytoin can be altered by disease and drug interactions that further complicate interpretation of plasma levels.

Dose

Loading Dose

- ⇨ Usual loading dose:
    - □ adults: 15 mg/kg
    - □ children (6 mon–6 yr): 15 mg/kg
    - □ children (0–3 mon): 15–20 mg/kg

- ⇨ Loading dose also can be calculated based upon the Cp desired:

$$\text{Loading Dose} = \frac{(Vd)(Cp)}{(S)(F)} \qquad \text{(Eq 11, pg 19)}$$

⇨ Oral loading doses >400 mg should be administered in multiple daily divided doses. For example, a 900 mg oral loading dose could be administered by giving 300 mg initially, followed by 300 mg Q 2 hr until the full 900 mg is administered.

⇨ Splitting the loading dose decreases the incidence of nausea and vomiting, increases patient's acceptance. Slow absorption causes the time to peak plasma concentration to be delayed.

⇨ Intravenous loading doses should not be administered at a rate >50 mg/min because of possible cardiovascular collapse and central nervous system (CNS) depression associated with the diluent, propylene glycol. Vital signs should be monitored throughout the infusion.

Maintenance Dose

⇨ Adults: 5–7 mg/kg/day.

⇨ Children (6 mon–6 yr): 5–15 mg/kg/day.

⇨ Children (0–3 mon): 3–5 mg/kg/day.

Therapeutic & Toxic Range

Therapeutic Range

⇨ 10–20 mg/L.

⇨ Assumes normal protein binding.

Toxic Concentrations

Table 10.1 **Therapeutic and Toxic Plasma Concentrations**

	Concentration (mg/L)
Sub Therapeutic	<5
Therapeutic	10–20
Toxic	15–30
Toxic	>30

Table 10.2 **Adverse Effects**

	Dose (mg/L)	*Concentration Related*	*Nonconcentration Related*
Sub Therapeutic	>5	None usually observed	Cardiovascular collapse and CNS depression when drug is administered IV too rapidly. **Do not** exceed 50 mg/min when infusing.[a]
Therapeutic	10–20	None usually observed	• Gingival hyperplasia • Folate deficiency anemia • Carbohydrate intolerance • Peripheral neuropathy • Thickening of facial features
Toxic	>30	• Nystagmus (15–30 mg/L) • Ataxia, lethargy • Vertigo • Decreased mental capacity	

[a]Problems secondary to propylene glycol.

Pharmacokinetic Parameters

Bioavailability (F)

Table 10.3

	Bioavailability (F)
IV	1.0
Oral	1.0
IM	Erratic: may require up to 5 days for complete absorption; crystallizes at intramuscular pH; not recommended

Table 10.4	**Time To Peak Plasma Concentration (Dilantin Kapseals)[a]**	
	Dose (mg)	Peak Time (hr)
	400	8.4
	800	13.2
	1600	31.5

[a]Chewable tabs and suspensions may peak within 1–3 hr.

⇨ *Factors altering absorption:*

- □ nasogastric (NG) feedings: continuous NG feedings can dramatically decrease the bioavailability (patients may require as much as 1200 mg/day)

- □ bioavailability may be improved by discontinuing NG feedings for 1–2 hr before and after medication administration

- □ increased gut motility can decrease bioavailability

⇨ Generic brand substitution is not recommended.

Table 10.5 **Salt Fraction (S)**

Dosage Form	Drug Amount	Salt Fraction (S)
Sodium phenytoin injectable	50 mg/mL	0.92
Sodium phenytoin capsule	30 mg	0.92
Sodium phenytoin capsule	100 mg	0.92
Phenytoin capsule (chewable)	50 mg	1.0
Phenyoin pediatric suspension[a]	30 mg/5 mL	1.0
Phenytoin suspension[a]	125 mg/5 mL	1.0

[a]Shake well. Care should be taken when measuring doses of the suspension; small changes in dose can result in large alterations in plasma concentration.

Volume of Distribution (Vd)

⇨ Vd = 0.65 L/kg.

⇨ Difficult to assess.

⇨ Roughly equivalent to total body water.

⇨ Distribution is complete at ≈60 min following an IV dose.

⇨ Consider only one compartment for oral doses.

⇨ Affected by albumin; decreased albumin (or binding) results in an increased Vd.

Clearance (Cl) & Half-Life (t½)

$$Cl_{phenytoin} = \frac{Vm}{Km + Cpss\ ave}$$

⇨ Cl is concentration dependent and is not a useful term in the clinical evaluation of phenytoin kinetics. The process appears to be first-order when Cpss is small compared to Michaelis-Menten constant (Km). In this situation, Cl is approximately equal to Vm/Km.

⇨ When Cpss approaches or exceeds Km, the Cl decreases resulting in a disproportionate increase in Cpss with each dosage increment. Cl may be calculated from the above equation but is of limited value.

⇨ Half-life (t½): The usual range is 20–24 hr. t½ is not constant because it increases with concentration.

⇨ Km:

  ▫ adults: 4 mg/L

  ▫ children (6 mon–16 yr): 7 mg/L

⇨ Vm:

  ▫ adults: 7 mg/kg/day

  ▫ children (7–16 yr): 8–10 mg/kg/day

  ▫ children (6 mon–6 yr): 10–13 mg/kg/day

Useful Pharmacokinetic Equations

Loading Dose

$$\text{Loading Dose} = \frac{(Vd)(Cp)}{(S)(F)}$$

(Eq 11, pg 19)

Maintenance Dose

$$(S)(F)(\text{Dose}/\tau) = \frac{(Vm)(Cpss\ ave)}{Km + Cpss\ ave}$$

(Eq 10.5, pg 318)

Steady-State Concentration

$$\text{Cpss} = \frac{(Km)[(S)(F)(Dose/\tau)]}{Vm - [(S)(F)(Dose/\tau)]} \quad \text{(Eq 10.6, pg 318)}$$

Adjustment for Serum Albumin (Cl$_{Cr}$ >25 mL/min)

$$\text{Cp}_{\text{Normal Binding}} = \frac{Cp'}{(1 - \alpha)\left[\dfrac{P'}{P_{NL}}\right] + \alpha} \quad \text{(Pg 314)}$$

⇨ *Note:* Normal serum albumin = 4.4 gm/dL.

Adjustment for Serum Albumin (Cl$_{Cr}$ <10 mL/min)

$$\text{Cp}_{\text{Normal Binding}} = \frac{Cp'}{(0.48)(1 - \alpha)\left[\dfrac{P'}{P_{NL}}\right] + \alpha} \quad \text{(Eq 10.2, pg 315)}$$

Mass Balance Equations

⇨ For an explanation of mass balance, please see **Basic Clinical Pharmacokinetics**, 3rd edition.[1]

$$\frac{\text{Amount Eliminated}}{t} = (S)(F)(Dose/\tau) - \left[\frac{(Cp_2 - Cp_1)(Vd)}{t}\right] \quad \text{(Eq 10.21, pg 333)}$$

$$\frac{\left[\dfrac{\text{Amount Eliminated}}{t}\right]\left[Km + \left(\dfrac{Cp_1 + Cp_2}{2}\right)\right]}{\left(\dfrac{Cp_1 + Cp_2}{2}\right)} \quad \text{(Eq 10.22, pg 334)}$$

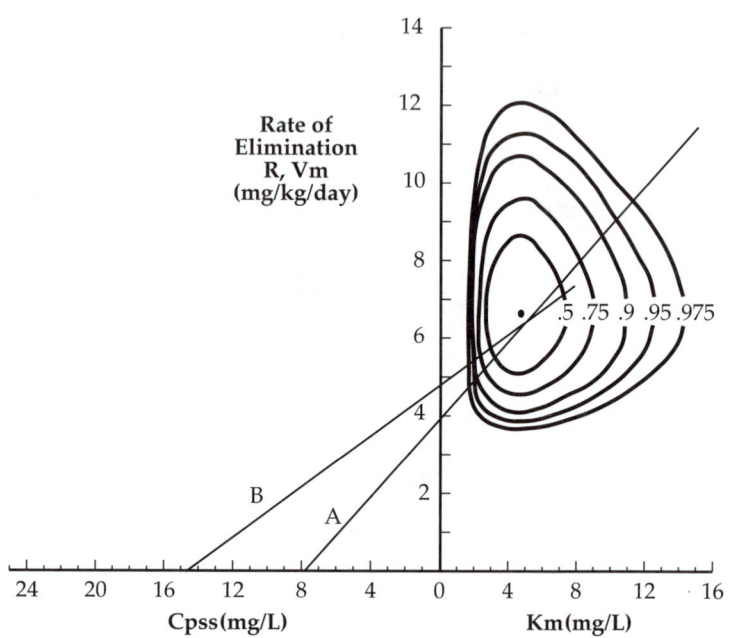

Figure 10.1. Orbit Graph: The most probable values of Vm and Km for a patient may be estimated using a single steady-state phenytoin concentration and a known dosing regimen. The concentric circles or "orbits" represent the fraction of the sample patient population whose Km and Vm values are within that orbit. 1) Plot the daily dose of phenytoin (mg/kg/day) on the vertical line (rate of elimination). 2) Plot the steady-state concentration (Cpss) on the horizontal line. 3) Draw a straight line connecting Cpss and daily dose through the orbits (line A). 4) The coordinates of the midpoint of the line crossing the innermost orbit through which the line passes are the most probable values for the patient's Vm and Km. 5) To calculate a new maintenance dose, draw a line from the point determined in Step 4 to the new desired Cpss' (line B). The point at which line B crosses the vertical line (rate of elimination) is the new maintenance dose (mg/kg/day). The line A represents a Cpss of 8 mg/L on 276 mg/day of phenytoin acid (300 mg/day of sodium phenytoin) for a 70 kg steady-state concentration was 15 mg/L (μg/mL). The original figure is modified so that R and Vm are in mg/kg/day of phenytoin acid. Reprinted with permission from reference 2.

Orbit Graph

⇨ For a detailed explanation of the orbit graph, see **Basic Clinical Pharmacokinetics**, 3rd edition.[1]

Serum Sampling Strategies

⇨ Trough levels are generally recommended. Cpss ave concentrations can be estimated from troughs in patients who are receiving oral or IV doses.

Oral

$$\text{Cpss ave} = [\text{Cpss min}] + \left[(0.25) \frac{(S)(F)(Dose)}{Vd} \right]$$

(Eq 10.17, pg 326)

IV

$$\text{Cpss ave} = [\text{Cpss min}] + \left[(0.5) \frac{(S)(F)(Dose)}{Vd} \right]$$

(Eq 10.16, pg 326)

⇨ Phenytoin concentration usually should be measured:

- □ after loading dose
- □ 2–3 days following initiation of therapy and again 6–7 days later
- □ every 3–12 months after steady state has been achieved
- □ in the presence of seizure activity
- □ in the presence of possible toxicity

☐ after the addition or deletion of medications that are known inhibitors or inducers of phenytoin metabolism

⇨ The time to reach steady state with phenytoin depends upon the patient's Km, Vm, and the dose of medication being administered. The following equation may be used to determine the time required to reach 90% of steady state. This equation assumes the patient's initial concentration is zero; however, it may be used in situations where the concentration is greater than zero, but less than the desired steady-state concentration.

$$t_{90\%} = \frac{(Km)(Vd)}{[Vm - (S)(F)(Dose/day)]^2} [(2.3\ Vm) - (0.9)(S)(F)(Dose/day)]$$

(Eq 10.13, pg 323)

Dialyzability

Hemodialysis

⇨ Not removed.

Peritoneal

⇨ Not removed.

Monitoring Parameters

Subjective

⇨ Drowsiness.

⇨ Fatigue.

Objective

⇨ Nystagmus.

⇨ Seizure activity.

⇨ Serum albumin.

⇨ Periodontal examination.

⇨ Ataxia.

⇨ Renal function.

⇨ Phenytoin plasma concentrations.

⇨ Complete blood count (CBC).

Drug Interactions

⇨ *Carbamazepine.* Phenytoin may induce the hepatic metabolism of this drug.

⇨ *Chloramphenicol* may increase the plasma concentration of phenytoin. Phenytoin may induce the hepatic metabolism of this medication, reducing its effectiveness.

⇨ *Cimetidine* may increase the plasma concentration of phenytoin.

⇨ *Corticosteroids.* Phenytoin may induce the hepatic metabolism of this medication, reducing its effectiveness.

⇨ *Cyclosporine.* Phenytoin may induce the hepatic metabolism of this medication, reducing its effectiveness.

⇨ *Dicumerol* may increase the plasma concentration of phenytoin.

⇨ *Disopyramide.* Phenytoin may induce the hepatic metabolism of this medication, reducing its effectiveness.

⇨ *Disulfiram* may increase the plasma concentration of phenytoin.

⇨ *Doxycycline.* Phenytoin may induce the hepatic metabolism of this medication, reducing its effectiveness.

⇨ *Ethosuxamide.* Phenytoin may induce the hepatic metabolism of this drug.

⇨ *Isoniazid* may increase the plasma concentration of phenytoin. This interaction may be canceled out by the concomitant use of rifampin.

⇨ *Meperidine.* Phenytoin may induce the hepatic metabolism of this medication, reducing its effectiveness.

⇨ *Methadone.* Phenytoin may induce the hepatic metabolism of this medication, reducing its effectiveness.

⇨ *Mexiletine.* Phenytoin may induce the hepatic metabolism of this medication, reducing its effectiveness.

⇨ *Oral contraceptives.* Phenytoin may induce the hepatic metabolism of this medication, reducing its effectiveness.

⇨ *Phenobarbital.* Phenytoin may induce the hepatic metabolism of this drug. Conversely, phenobarbital may induce the metabolism of phenytoin.

⇨ *Phenylbutazone* may displace phenytoin from plasma protein binding sites; however, unbound concentrations of phenytoin remain relatively unchanged.

⇨ *Primidone.* Phenytoin may induce the hepatic metabolism of this drug.

⇨ *Quinidine.* Phenytoin may induce the hepatic metabolism of this medication, reducing its effectiveness.

⇨ *Rifampin* may decrease the plasma concentration of phenytoin (interaction may be canceled out by the concomitant use of isoniazid). Phenytoin may induce the hepatic metabolism of this medication, reducing its effectiveness.

⇨ *Salicylates* may displace phenytoin from plasma protein binding sites; however, unbound concentrations of phenytoin remain relatively unchanged.

⇨ *Sulfonamides* may increase the plasma concentration of phenytoin.

⇨ *Theophylline.* Phenytoin may induce the hepatic metabolism of this medication, reducing its effectiveness.

⇨ *Tolbutamide* may displace phenytoin from plasma protein binding sites; however, unbound concentrations of phenytoin remain relatively unchanged.

⇨ *Trimethoprim* may increase the plasma concentration of phenytoin.

⇨ *Valproic acid.* Phenytoin may induce the hepatic metabolism of this drug. Valproic acid may inhibit the metabolism of phenytoin, and displace phenytoin from protein binding sites.

⇨ *Warfarin.* Phenytoin may induce the hepatic metabolism of this medication, reducing its effectiveness.

Special Considerations for IV Administration

⇨ Phenytoin never should be administered IV at a rate exceeding 50 mg/min.

⇨ *Compatibilities.* Should be diluted in a small quantity of 0.45% or 0.9% normal saline (NS) at a concentration of 20–30 mg/mL and administered immediately upon preparation. The solution should be observed for crystal formation. Some clinicians recommend using an in-line filter.

⇨ *Incompatibilities.* Phenytoin should not be mixed with other medications or injected into a Y-site with other medications because immediate precipitation often occurs.

References

1. Winter ME. Basic Clinical Pharmacokinetics. 3rd ed. Vancouver: Applied Therapeutics; 1994;312–348.

2. Winter ME, Tozer TN. Phenytoin. In: Evans WE et al., eds. Applied Pharmacokinetics: Principles of Therapeutic Drug Monitoring. 3rd ed. Vancouver: Applied Therapeutics; 1992;1-25-1-44.

3. Choonara IA, Rane A. Therapeutic Monitoring of Anticonvulsants, state of the art. Clin Pharmacokinet. 1990;18(4):318–328.

Primidone 11

Primidone is an anticonvulsant that is structurally similar to phenobarbital. The parent drug itself is active and is metabolized by the liver to active compounds; one of these compounds is phenobarbital. For this reason, many individuals view primidone as a prodrug of phenobarbital. When monitoring plasma drug concentrations, it is necessary to consider both primidone and phenobarbital concentrations. An adequate understanding of the pharmacokinetic disposition of both primidone and its metabolite is critical since there are notable differences in the elimination half-life of these two drugs.

Dose

Loading Dose

> ⇨ None required.

Maintenance Dose

> ⇨ Approximately ⅕ of primidone is metabolized to phenobarbital; therefore, the recommended dose of primidone is roughly 5 times greater than that of phenobarbital.

> ⇨ *General dosing guidelines:*
> > □ adults: 10–20 mg/kg/day
> > □ children: 15–30 mg/kg/day

> ⇨ Therapy should be initiated at a low dose and long interval and gradually adjusted upward.

⇨ A common schedule used to initiate primidone is as follows:

  □ 100–125 mg Q HS for days 1–3
  □ 100–125 mg ↑ BID for days 4–6
  □ 100–125 mg ↑ TID for days 7–9
  □ ↑ 125–250 mg TID
  □ *note:* break a 250 mg tablet in half to obtain 125 mg dose

⇨ After stabilized on a specific regimen, any dosage change should result in a proportional change in the plasma concentration (unlike carbamazepine).

Therapeutic & Toxic Range

Therapeutic Range

⇨ 5–12 mg/L.

Toxic Concentrations

⇨ >15 mg/L.

⇨ **Side effects** encountered are similar to those with phenobarbital:

  □ sedation (barbiturate)
  □ ataxia
  □ nystagmus
  □ nausea and vomiting
  □ respiratory depression (overdose)
  □ dermatologic problems

⇨ Toxicity may be minimized by gradually increasing the dose over time.

Pharmacokinetic Parameters

Bioavailability (F)

⇨ Only available in oral dosage formulations:
- □ tablets: 50 and 250 mg
- □ suspension: 250 mg/5 mL

⇨ Absorption appears to be fairly complete (F = 0.8–1.0).

⇨ Peak plasma concentrations are achieved 1–4 hr after an oral dose.

⇨ Primidone is not formulated as a salt (S = 1.0).

Volume of Distribution (Vd)

⇨ Average Vd = 0.6 L/kg (wide range: 0.4–1.14 L/kg).

⇨ Protein binding is minimal (<20%) which allows for adequate distribution into cerebrospinal fluid (CSF).

Clearance (Cl) & Half-Life (t½)

⇨ 80% is metabolized by the liver:
- □ 60% to a mildly active phenylethylmalonamide (PEMA)
- □ 20% to phenobarbital

⇨ Remaining 20% is excreted unchanged in the urine.

⇨ Cl should consider both hepatic and renal elimination:
- □ $Cl_{hepatic} = 0.06$ L/kg/hr
- □ $Cl_{renal} = 0.015$ L/kg/hr
- □ $Cl_{primidone \rightarrow phenobarb} = 0.012$ L/kg/hr

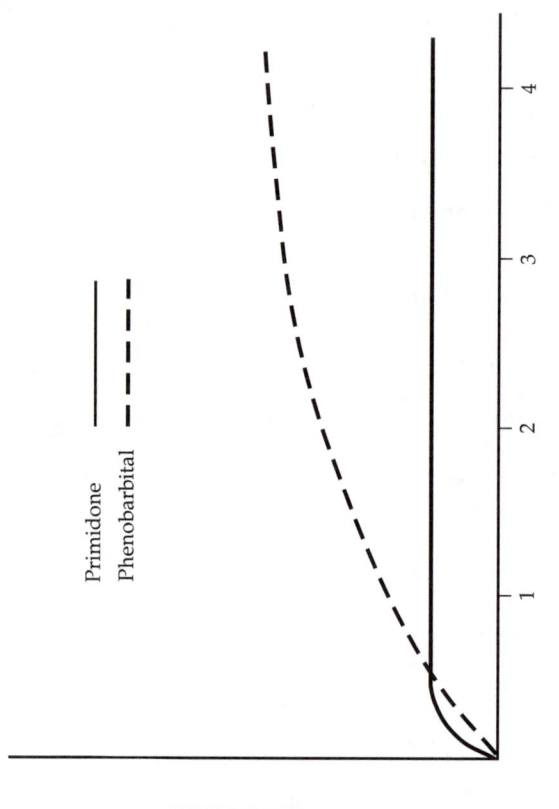

Figure 11.1. Phenobarbital Concentrations Derived from Primidone. During the first few days to weeks after starting primidone therapy, primidone and phenobarbital plasma concentrations are similar. As steady state is approached, the phenobarbital level is approximately 2 to 4 times greater than the primidone concentration.

⇨ $t\frac{1}{2}$ = 8 hr (range: 4–15 hr).

  □ requires a more frequent dosing interval than phenobarbital

  □ reaches steady state significantly earlier than phenobarbital (see Serum Sampling Strategies)

Serum Sampling Strategies

⇨ Both primidone and phenobarbital plasma concentrations must be evaluated.

⇨ Steady state will be reached much earlier for primidone (1–2 days) compared to phenobarbital (3–4 weeks).

⇨ The full anticonvulsant effect is not observed until steady states for both parent drug and metabolite are reached.

⇨ Upward adjustments in the dosing regimen before steady state may result in elevated plasma concentrations and toxicity.

⇨ Due to the shorter $t\frac{1}{2}$ of primidone, plasma concentrations should be sampled at a consistent time; usually just before the subsequent dose (trough).

Dialyzability

Hemodialysis & Peritoneal

⇨ Like phenobarbital, primidone is removed by hemodialysis and peritoneal dialysis; however, the extent of removal is unclear.

Monitoring Parameters

Subjective

⇨ Altered mentation.

⇨ Seizure control or seizure frequency.

⇨ Compliance.

Objective

⇨ Primidone plasma concentrations.

⇨ Phenobarbital plasma concentrations.

⇨ Vital signs.

⇨ White blood cell (WBC) count.

⇨ Platelets.

⇨ Electroencephalogram (EEG).

Drug Interactions

⇨ Because of its conversion to phenobarbital, primidone can interact with the same drugs as phenobarbital (see Phenobarbital on page 130).

⇨ *Carbamazepine* can enhance the conversion of primidone to phenobarbital through the induction of hepatic enzymes.

⇨ *Phenytoin* can enhance the conversion of primidone to phenobarbital through the induction of hepatic enzymes.

⇨ *Valproic acid.* When used concurrently, valproic acid can increase primidone plasma concentrations due to competitive inhibition of hepatic enzymes. Phenobarbital concentrations also can be influenced by the decreased conversion or metabolism of primidone into phenobarbital.

Special Considerations

⇨ The use of primidone in combination with phenobarbital is discouraged to minimize the possibility of excess phenobarbital plasma concentrations.

References

1. Winter ME. Basic Clinical Pharmacokinetics. 3rd ed. Vancouver: Applied Therapeutics; 1994:349–355.

Notes:

Procainamide   12

Procainamide, a type IA antiarrhythmic agent, is used to manage patients with ventricular and atrial arrhythmias. Although procainamide is effective, its short half-life necessitates frequent dosing or the use of sustained-release formulations. The drug-induced systemic lupus erythematosus (SLE) associated with its use also is of concern.

The pharmacokinetic disposition of procainamide varies considerably between patients. Patients have a genetic predisposition to be fast or slow acetylators and the drug is eliminated by both hepatic and renal mechanisms.

Dose

Loading Dose

Similar to lidocaine, procainamide's volume of distribution has two distinct compartments: an initial compartment (Vi) into which an IV dose initially distributes, and a much larger tissue compartment (Vd) into which the majority (70%) of the dose is distributed over time. When calculating an IV loading dose of procainamide, it is important to consider the total amount of drug needed to "fill" both the initial and tissue compartments; however, this dose must be administered over a long enough period to allow ample time for distribution into the larger tissue compartment.

⇨ One strategy involves calculating the appropriate total loading dose required (based upon Vd).

▫ administer ≈30% initially (which corresponds to Vi)

- □ follow the initial dose with subsequent "mini-boluses" at 15–20 min intervals

- □ repeat "mini-boluses" until the patient responds, side effects are encountered, or the total loading dose is given

⇨ The loading dose is based upon ideal body weight (IBW) because very little procainamide distributes into adipose tissue.

Maintenance Dose

⇨ A maintenance infusion usually is started after the loading dose to maintain the desired plasma concentration.

⇨ In contrast to the loading dose, the maintenance infusion usually is based upon the patient's actual body weight.

⇨ Oral regimens are limited to the dosage strengths in available formulations making it more difficult to achieve a specific serum level; however, in most situations an optimal dosage regimen can be determined.

⇨ The two-compartment Vd is not as critical to consider for oral regimens because absorption period is prolonged.

⇨ The total daily oral dose usually is calculated and given in divided doses based upon the specific formulation used.

- □ immediate release products (Pronestyl): dosed Q 3–4 hr

- □ sustained release products (Procan-SR): dosed Q 6–8 hr

□ immediate release agents may be used initially to achieve more rapid plasma concentrations

⇨ *General dosing guidelines:*

□ total IV loading dose = 17 mg/kg (IBW)

  ○ give as divided doses at 15–20 min intervals or slowly over at least 1 hr

  ○ use a total dose of 12 mg/kg in patients with Cl_{Cr} <20 mL/min

□ IV maintenance infusion ≈2.8 mg/kg/hr (actual body weight)

  ○ reduce in patients with compromised renal function

□ oral maintenance dose ≈50 mg/kg/day given in divided doses

Therapeutic & Toxic Range

Plasma concentrations of both procainamide (PA) and its primary metabolite, N-acetylprocainamide (NAPA) frequently are monitored to assess efficacy and toxicity. Procainamide concentrations tend to be a more useful indicator of efficacy, and NAPA levels are more helpful to monitor toxicity. In patients with impaired renal function, NAPA accumulates to a greater extent than PA because NAPA depends upon renal function for elimination to a greater extent than PA.

Therapeutic Concentrations

⇨ Procainamide: 4–8 mg/L (up to 10–12 mg/L for refractory arrhythmias).

⇨ NAPA: 10–20 mg/L.

Toxic Concentrations

⮑ Procainamide >12 mg/L.

⮑ NAPA >25–30 mg/L.

⮑ Procainamide + NAPA >30 mg/L.

⮑ *Signs of toxicity:*
- □ GI intolerance
- □ weakness
- □ sweating
- □ malaise
- □ neutropenia
- □ hypotension
- □ bradycardia
- □ heart block
- □ prolonged electrocardiogram (ECG) intervals

⮑ Procainamide-induced SLE is associated to a greater extent with procainamide than NAPA.
- □ more common in slow versus fast acetylators (procainamide >NAPA)
- □ tends to occur with prolonged administration (>6–12 mon)

Pharmacokinetic Parameters

Bioavailability (F)

⮑ Available dosage forms include oral, IV and IM.
- □ immediate release: Pronestyl 250, 375, and 500 mg tablets

□ sustained release: Procan-SR 250, 500, 750, and 1000 mg wax matrix tablets

□ injection: 100 and 500 mg/mL

⇨ Oral products most frequently are utilized (F = 0.66–1.13; average = 0.85).

⇨ Peak concentrations occur 1–2 hr after Pronestyl and 3–4 hr after Procan-SR; food delays the rate but not extent of absorption.

⇨ Both oral products are available as the HCl salt (S = 0.87 procainamide).

⇨ IM procainamide injections peak after ≈25 min with fairly complete absorption.

Volume of Distribution (Vd)

⇨ Rapidly and widely distributed with 70% of procainamide bound to tissues.

⇨ Distribution characteristics similar to lidocaine.

⇨ Initially distributed into serum or initial compartment (Vi = 0.67 L/kg).

⇨ Volume greatly expands as procainamide is distributed into tissue compartment (Vd = 2.0 L/kg).

⇨ Congestive heart failure (CHF) will reduce both Vi and Vd by ≈25% (Vi = 0.5 L/kg; Vd = 1.5 L/kg).

⇨ Distribution into the tissues usually is complete within 20–30 min ($t\frac{1}{2}\alpha$ = 5 min).

⇨ Only 15% procainamide is bound to proteins.

Clearance (Cl) & Half-Life (t½)

⇨ Approximately 50% of procainamide is metabolized by the liver and the remaining 50% is excreted renally.

⇨ Primary metabolic pathway involves acetylation to NAPA.

  □ acetylation mostly occurs in liver, but also can occur in the lungs, kidney, red blood cells

  □ additional metabolites include DEPA (desethylation) and PABA (hydrolysis)

⇨ Two genetic predispositions exist: fast acetylator and slow acetylator phenotypes.

  □ Caucasians and blacks have an equal probability of being either fast or slow acetylators

  □ Asians and Eskimos tend to be predominantly fast acetylators (80%–90%)

⇨ Acetylator status is determined by NAPA:procainamide ratio:

  □ ratios are only for patients with normal renal function; decreased renal function results in an increase in the NAPA:procainamide ratio

	NAPA:procainamide
Fast acetylator	>1.2:1
Slow acetylator	<0.8:1

⇨ Procainamide Cl must consider contributions of the liver ($Cl_{acetylation}$), kidneys (Cl_{renal}) and other (Cl_{other}).

  □ $Cl_{acetylation}$ is dependent upon acetylator status:

- fast$_{ace}$: Cl = 0.19 L/kg/hr (3.2 mL/kg/min)
- slow$_{ace}$: Cl = 0.07 L/kg/hr (1.1 mL/kg/min)
- ave$_{ace}$: Cl = 0.13 L/kg/hr (2.2 mL/kg/min)
- Cl_{renal} = Cl_{Cr} mL/min × 3
- Cl_{other} = 0.10 L/kg/hr (1.66 mL/kg/min)

⇨ Factors that decrease procainamide Cl:
- chronic liver disease
- CHF (↓ perfusion)
- impaired renal function
- advanced age

⇨ t½ of procainamide = 3–5 hr.

⇨ t½ of NAPA = 5–8 hr.

Useful Pharmacokinetic Equations

Initial Loading Dose (see pg 154)

$$\text{Initial Loading Dose} = \frac{(Vi)(Cp\ max\ desired)}{(S)(F)}$$

Total Loading Dose (see pg 154)

$$\text{Total Loading Dose} = \frac{(Vd)(Cp\ max\ desired)}{(S)(F)}$$

Maintenance Dose

$$\text{Maintenance Dose} = \frac{(Cl_{total})(Cpss\ ave)(\tau)}{(S)(F)}$$

Switching from IV to an Equivalent Oral Dose

$$\text{Daily Oral Dose} \atop \text{(mg)} = \frac{\left(\dfrac{Cp_{oral}}{Cp_{IV}}\right)\left(\substack{\text{infusion rate} \\ \text{(mg/hr)}}\right)\left(24 \text{ hr/day}\right)}{(F)}$$

Note: If the oral concentration desired is the same as Cp_{IV}, the term, $\dfrac{Cp_{oral}}{Cp_{IV}}$ can be eliminated from the equation.

Serum Sampling Strategies

⇨ Procainamide plasma concentrations usually are obtained to assess efficacy.

⇨ NAPA concentrations more often are used to assess toxicity.

⇨ For patients on IV procainamide infusions, sample after steady state ($\approx$12–24 hr).

⇨ For patients receiving oral regimens, draw steady-state serum samples just before a dose (trough) to avoid the considerable variations associated with oral absorption.

⇨ Prompt handling of serum samples is necessary to avoid potential *in vitro* metabolism by red blood cells.

Dialyzability

Hemodialysis. The fairly low molecular weight and minimal protein binding of procainamide results in significant removal of both procainamide and NAPA by hemodialysis. Supplemental procainamide doses may be necessary depending upon the duration of the dialysis run.

Peritoneal. Procainamide does not appear to be effectively removed by peritoneal dialysis.

Monitoring Parameters

Subjective

> ⇨ Fatigue.

> ⇨ GI complaints.

Objective

> ⇨ Close ECG monitoring.

> ⇨ Procainamide plasma concentrations.

> ⇨ Vital signs.

> ⇨ White blood cell (WBC) count with differential.

> ⇨ Platelets.

> ⇨ SLE symptoms.

> ⇨ Positive ANA titers (antinuclear antibody).

Drug Interactions

> ⇨ *Other cardiovascular agents.* Procainamide can potentiate the effect of other antiarrhythmic and hypotensive agents and can cause pronounced hypotension or slowing of conduction.

> ⇨ *Cimetidine and ranitidine* reduce the Cl of procainamide by inhibiting tubular secretion. Cimetidine interferes to a greater extent than ranitidine (43% versus 20% Cl reduction, respectively).

⇨ *Anticholinergic agents.* Procainamide possesses anticholinergic properties which can potentiate the effect of other anticholinergics. In addition, procainamide should be avoided in patients with myasthenia gravis due to the likelihood of procainamide blocking the effects of cholinesterase inhibitors and worsening the myasthenia gravis.

⇨ *Phenytoin and phenobarbital.* The enzyme inducing ability of these anticonvulsants can potentially enhance the elimination of procainamide; however, the clinical significance of this interaction is questionable.

Special Considerations

⇨ The infusion rate of IV procainamide should not exceed 50 mg/min. Significant hypotension and additional adverse reactions are more likely to occur if the rate of infusion is >50 mg/min.

⇨ Mixtures of IV procainamide and dextrose (concentration of 1 mg/mL D5W) have resulted in a 12% loss of active drug over a 24-hr period at room temperature. Therefore, IV preparations of procainamide mixed in D5W should be administered within 8–12 hr after preparation or mixed in normal saline.

⇨ Additional physical incompatibilities have been reported with parenteral procainamide when mixed with some drugs. For more information regarding specific drug compatibilities see a detailed reference.

⇨ Procan-SR is formulated in a wax matrix that may be excreted intact in the feces. The patient should be assured that this is normal and the active drug has been absorbed.

References

1. Winter ME. Basic Clinical Pharmacokinetics. 3rd ed. Vancouver: Applied Therapeutics; 1994:356–378.

2. Coyle JD, Lima JJ. Procainamide. In: Evans WE et al., eds. Applied Pharmacokinetics: Principles of Therapeutic Drug Monitoring. 3rd ed. Vancouver: Applied Therapeutics; 1992:22-1–22-33.

3. Trissel LA. Handbook of Injectable Drugs. 6th ed. Bethesda: American Society of Hospital Pharmacists; 1990.

4. King JC. Guide to Parenteral Admixtures. St Louis: Pacemarq, Inc; 1994.

Notes:

Quinidine   13

Type IA antiarrhythmic agents such as procainamide, disopyramide, and quinidine share several similar characteristics. However, toxicities associated with the use of quinidine, particularly
diarrhea and other GI complaints, tend to limit its utility. Individ-
ualizing quinidine therapy is justified by factors such as its narrow
therapeutic index, the considerable interpatient variability that exists with the drug, the multitude of available quinidine formulations, and the drug and disease state factors that can significantly
affect the pharmacokinetics of quinidine.

Dose

Because of the large degree of patient variability that exists with
quinidine, general mg/kg dosing recommendations must be used
cautiously and only as a general guide. Accurate calculations
which take into consideration patient specific clearance should be
used to arrive at a more appropriate dosage regimen.

⇨ Quinidine is similar to lidocaine in regard to its two-
   compartment characteristics.

⇨ Primary use of oral, rather than IV route, places less
   emphasis on Vi and Vd; instead, calculations are based
   upon the desired Cpss ave and quinidine Cl.

⇨ *General guidelines for daily oral doses:*

   ☐ dose ranges:

      ○ quinidine sulfate: 800–2400 mg/day

      ○ quinidine gluconate: 660–2970 mg/day

   ☐ 18–20 mg/kg/day of quinidine base also has
      been used

- □ daily doses are divided into equal doses and given:
  - ○ Q 4–6 hr for conventional, immediate-release products
  - ○ Q 8–12 hr for sustained-release (SR) formulations
- □ congestive heart failure (CHF) may cause a 25% reduction in the daily dose requirement

⇨ IV dosage regimens rarely are used:
- □ 500 mg quinidine gluconate in 50 mL D5W administered slowly over 30–60 min

Therapeutic & Toxic Range

⇨ The specific assay method used must be considered when evaluating quinidine plasma concentrations. The more sensitive the assay [e.g., high-performance liquid chromatography (HPLC)], the lower the reported serum samples and therapeutic range (for further explanation, see **Basic Clinical Pharmacokinetics**, 3rd edition).[1]

⇨ Quinidine plasma concentrations correlate reasonably well with therapeutic response and toxicity.

Therapeutic Concentrations

⇨ 2–5 mg/L (double extraction assay).

⇨ If maximal concentrations fail to evoke a therapeutic response, do not push any higher; choose an alternative agent.

Toxic Concentrations

⇨ Toxicity appears to be dose-dependent.

⇨ Tends to occur at concentrations >10 mg/L.

⇨ *Toxic symptoms:*

  ◻ GI complaints are the most common (diarrhea, nausea, vomiting) and often result in discontinuation; gluconate formulations may be better tolerated than sulfate products

  ◻ cinchonism

  ◻ bradycardia

  ◻ heart block

  ◻ hypotension

  ◻ drug fever

  ◻ hypersensitivity reactions

Pharmacokinetic Parameters

Bioavailability (F)

  ⇨ Quinidine is available in several different dosage formulations:

Formulation	Available Strengths
Quinidine sulfate	Cin-Quin 100, 200, and 300 mg Quinora 200 and 300 mg Quinidex (SR) 300 mg Injectable (200 mg/mL)
Quinidine gluconate	Quinaglute (SR) 324 mg Duraquin (SR) 330 mg Injectable (50 mg/mL)
Quinidine polygalacturonate	Cardioquin 275 mg (equivalent to 200 mg quinidine SO_4)

⇨ Oral bioavailability can vary considerably (F for SO_4 = 0.73; F for gluconate = 0.70).

⇨ Peak concentrations after oral doses occur in 1–3 hr (up to 5 hr for SR products).

⇨ Food delays the rate of absorption; antacids and anti-diarrheal agents can delay the extent of absorption.

⇨ Salt forms (S):

  □ sulfate = 0.82

  □ gluconate = 0.62

  □ polygalacturonate = 0.62

⇨ Oral products are used most frequently; IV quinidine is used rarely (if IV needed, use procainamide).

⇨ IM route should be avoided because of the severe pain and muscle damage associated with the injections and erratic and incomplete absorption.

Volume of Distribution (Vd)

⇨ Very rapid and extensive distribution.

⇨ 70%–90% is bound to protein (primarily to α-1-acid glycoprotein).

⇨ Factors that affect protein binding may alter quinidine disposition (see **Basic Clinical Pharmacokinetics**, 3rd edition for more information).[1]

⇨ Vi = 1.0 L/kg; Vd = 2.7 L/kg.

⇨ Characteristic two-compartment distribution, but Vd is used to calculate dosage regimens.

⇨ Additional factors may influence the distribution of quinidine:

	Vi (L/kg)	Vd (L/kg)
Normal	1.0	2.7
CHF	—	↓ 1.8
Cirrhosis	—	↑ 3.8

Clearance (Cl) & Half-Life (t½)

⇨ 80% of quinidine is metabolized by the liver and only 10%–20% is renally excreted.

⇨ Unclear what role the metabolites play in either efficacy or toxicity.

⇨ Quinidine:

▫ Cl = 0.28 L/kg/hr (4.7 mL/kg/min)

▫ Cl_{CHF} = 0.20 L/kg/hr (3.3 mL/kg/min)

⇨ t½ = 6–7 hr (not significantly prolonged by decreased renal function).

Useful Pharmacokinetic Equations

Initial Oral Dose

$$\text{Oral dose}/24\ hr = \frac{(Cl)(Cpss\ ave)}{(S)(F)}$$

Serum Sampling Strategies

⇨ Steady state occurs after ≈2 days (28–35 hr).

⇨ Concentrations may be obtained before steady state if toxicity is suspected.

⇨ Obtain trough concentrations to avoid variability associated with peak concentrations.

⇨ Serum quinidine levels need not be routinely monitored.

⇨ Plasma concentrations are most helpful to assess patient compliance, drug-drug or drug-disease interactions.

Dialyzability

Hemodialysis & Peritoneal

⇨ Quinidine is poorly removed by hemodialysis and the drug is not removed by peritoneal dialysis.

Monitoring Parameters

Subjective

⇨ Diarrhea, nausea, vomiting.

⇨ Hypersensitivity reactions (i.e., rash).

⇨ Cinchonism (i.e., tinnitus, headache, visual disturbances).

Objective

⇨ Quinidine plasma concentrations.

⇨ Electrocardiogram (ECG).

⇨ Appearance of new arrhythmias.

⇨ White blood cell (WBC) count with differential.

Drug Interactions

⇨ *Amiodarone* can significantly decrease quinidine Cl.

⇨ *Anticholinergic agents.* The anticholinergic properties associated with quinidine can interfere with cholinesterase inhibitor treatment in patients with myasthenia gravis and worsen myasthenia gravis.

⇨ *Cimetidine* can significantly decrease quinidine Cl.

⇨ *Digoxin.* Quinidine significantly reduces both the Vd and Cl of digoxin resulting in a doubling of the digoxin concentration when quinidine is added. On the day quinidine therapy is implemented, skip the digoxin dose for that day and restart digoxin on the following day at 50% of the original dose.

⇨ *Other cardiovascular agents.* Quinidine can enhance the hypotensive and antiarrhythmic effects of other cardiovascular agents.

⇨ *Phenobarbital* induces metabolic enzymes and enhances quinidine Cl.

⇨ *Phenytoin* induces metabolic enzymes and enhances quinidine Cl.

⇨ *Rifampin* induces metabolic enzymes and enhances quinidine Cl.

Special Considerations

⇨ A rapid ventricular rate has been observed when quinidine is used to manage patients with atrial fibrillation. In this situation, treatment with digitalis before administration of quinidine will help to protect the ventricles from the rapid atrial rate.

References

1. Winter ME. Basic Clinical Pharmacokinetics. 3rd ed. Vancouver: Applied Therapeutics; 1994:379–395.

2. Ueda CT. Quinidine. In: Evans WE et al., eds. Applied Pharmacokinetics: Principles of Therapeutic Drug Monitoring. 3rd ed. Vancouver: Applied Therapeutics; 1992:23-1–23-22.

3. Crevasse L. Quinidine: an update on therapeutics, pharmacokinetics and serum drug monitoring. Am J Cardiol. 1988; 62:221–231.

Notes:

Salicylates 14

Salicylates have analgesic, antipyretic, and anti-inflammatory effects. The most frequently used salicylates include acetylsalicylic acid (aspirin), sodium salicylate, and choline chloride. These compounds are salts of the active drug, salicylic acid.

Salicylates inhibit prostaglandin (PG) synthesis by inhibiting the enzyme, cyclooxygenase, which is responsible for the conversion of arachidonic acid to two PG endoperoxides: PGG_2 and PGH_2. The inhibition of the production of PGG_2 and PGH_2 ultimately results in an attenuation of the usual end products, PGD_2 and PGE_2, which are responsible for vasodilation, enhanced pain, redness, and swelling. Low dose salicylates also reduce the production of platelet thromboxane A_2 (TXA_2) which results in a prolonged bleeding time. This action may prevent myocardial infarctions and cerebrovascular accidents, but also may be deleterious in patients with bleeding disorders or in patients being treated with other anticoagulants. Large doses of salicylates are required for anti-inflammatory activity. When anti-inflammatory doses are used, pharmacokinetic monitoring is indicated. Salicylates are metabolized by capacity-limited pathways and may accumulate to toxic concentrations, particularly when high doses are required.

Dose

Maintenance Dose (Anti-Inflammatory)

⇨ Adults: 45–60 mg/kg/day; given in 4–6 divided doses.

⇨ Children: 70–90 mg/kg/day; given in 4–6 divided doses.

Therapeutic & Toxic Range

Therapeutic Range

⇨ 100–300 mg/L (10–30 mg/dL).

Toxic Concentrations

Salicylate Level (mg/L)	Toxic Symptoms
<100	• Gastrointestinal intolerance • Gastrointestinal bleeding: may be circumvented with enteric coated aspirin or with the concurrent use of cimetidine
>200	• Headaches • Vertigo • Tinnitus • Deafness
>300–400	• Nausea • Vomiting
Overdose (500–900)	• Respiratory alkalosis • Metabolic acidosis • Fluid and electrolyte disturbances

⇨ *Allergic response (not concentration related):*

  ▫ renal dysfunction

  ▫ bronchospasm

  ▫ vasculitis

  ▫ serum sickness

  ▫ urticaria

  ▫ shock

Pharmacokinetic Parameters

Bioavailability (F)

⇨ Completely absorbed (F = 1.0).

⇨ Time to peak: 0.5–2 hr.

Compound	Salt Fraction (S)
Aspirin	0.77
Sodium salicylate	0.86
Magnesium salicylate	0.92
Choline magnesium salicylate	1.0[a]
Choline salicylate	0.56

[a]This product is labeled for salicylic acid content.

Volume of Distribution (Vd)

⇨ Varies with dose/concentration (see table below).

⇨ Governed by the availability of plasma protein binding sites. As binding sites are saturated, the Vd increases.

Plasma Concentration (mg/L)	Volume of Distribution (Vd) (L/kg)
<200	<0.2
200	0.2
>200	>0.2

Clearance (Cl) & Half-Life (t½).   The elimination of salicylates is very complex and occurs by multiple pathways: two capacity-limited metabolic pathways, two linear metabolic pathways, and one linear renal pathway. Saturable protein binding results in escalating free fractions as plasma concentrations are increased. The increased free fraction makes more of the drug available for metabolism. At concentrations between 100 and 300 mg/L, the capacity-limited metabolism and the saturable protein binding offset each other and the overall Cl is linear.

⇨ Cl = 0.012 L/kg/hr (within the therapeutic range).

⇨ t½ is extremely variable with salicylates (3–24 hr) and increases with plasma concentration.

Useful Pharmacokinetic Equations

Steady-State Concentrations

$$\text{Cpss ave} = \frac{(S)(F)(\text{Dose}/\tau)}{Cl} \qquad \text{(Eq 35, pg 46)}$$

Steady-State Trough Concentrations

$$\text{Cpss min} = \frac{\dfrac{(S)(F)(\text{Dose})}{Vd}}{(1 - e^{-Kd\tau})}(e^{-Kd\tau}) \qquad \text{(Eq 47, pg 55)}$$

Cpss min (Based Upon Cpss ave)

$$\text{Cpss min} = [\text{Cpss ave}] - \left[(0.5)\frac{(S)(F)(\text{Dose})}{Vd}\right] \qquad \text{(Eq 14.1, pg 402)}$$

Serum Sampling Strategies

⇨ Because of saturable protein binding, the most reproducible sampling time is just before a dose is given (trough).

⇨ The peak value can be predicted from the trough value.

⇨ The timing of the sample may not always be critical in the patient who is receiving anti-inflammatory doses of salicylates since the peak to trough difference may be negligible ($t\frac{1}{2} = 24$ hr, $\tau = 4$–6 hr which is $<\frac{1}{4}$ of $t\frac{1}{2}$).

⇨ The time required to reach steady state is quite variable with salicylates because $t\frac{1}{2}$ changes with concentrations.

⇨ Most clinicians consider one week to be a reasonable time to reach steady state in patients being treated with anti-inflammatory doses of salicylates.

Dialyzability

Hemodialysis: removed; dialysis clearance is extremely variable.

Hemoperfusion: removed; dialysis clearance is extremely variable.

Monitoring Parameters

Subjective

⇨ Pain.

⇨ Swelling.

⇨ Joint mobility.

⇨ Nausea and vomiting.

Objective

⇨ Signs of bleeding.

⇨ Erythrocyte sedimentation rate (ESR).

⇨ Tinnitus.

⇨ Vertigo.

Drug Interactions

⇨ *Ammonium chloride* decreases urinary Cl of salicylates.

⇨ *Antacids* increase urinary Cl of salicylates; have no effect on time to peak.

⇨ *Anticoagulants.* Salicylates may enhance the effects of oral anticoagulants.

⇨ *Antidepressants.* Salicylates increase plasma concentrations and toxicity of antidepressants.

⇨ *Corticosteroids* enhance renal Cl of salicylates.

⇨ *Ethanol* may enhance gastric toxicity.

⇨ *Food* increases time to peak of salicylates.

⇨ *Methotrexate.* Salicylates cause a prolonged elevation of unbound methotrexate, enhancing toxicity.

⇨ *Nonsteroidal anti-inflammatory drugs* may increase or decrease salicylate concentrations.

⮞ *Sulfonylureas.* Anti-inflammatory doses of salicylates may enhance the hypoglycemic activity of these agents.

⮞ *Uricosuric agents.* Salicylates at high doses may inhibit the uricosuric effect of these drugs. Sulfinpyrazone and probenecid may inhibit the uricosuric effect of salicylates.

References

1. Winter ME. Basic Clinical Pharmacokinetics. 3rd ed. Vancouver: Applied Therapeutics; 1994:396–404.

2. Dromgolle S, Furst D. Salicylates. In: Evans WE et al., eds. Applied Pharmacokinetics: Principles of Therapeutic Drug Monitoring. 3rd ed. Vancouver: Applied Therapeutics; 1992: 32-1–32-34.

3. McLeod D, Bailey J. Salicylates. In: Taylor W, Caviness M, eds. A Textbook for the Clinical Application of Therapeutic Drug Monitoring. Irving: Abbott Laboratories, Diagnostics Division; 1986:385–395.

Notes:

Theophylline 15

Theophylline is a xanthine derivative with a structure similar to caffeine and theobromine. It is used as a bronchodilator during acute asthmatic attacks and prophylactically to suppress symptoms of chronic airway disease. Theophylline also increases myocardial and diaphragmatic contractility and is used to treat Cheyne-Stokes respirations, neonatal idiopathic apnea, and bradycardia. Historically, theophylline was thought to act through inhibition of phosphodiesterase, leading to increased intracellular cAMP concentrations; however, concentrations required to cause phosphodiesterase inhibition are not attainable physiologically. Therefore, the precise mechanism of action of theophylline is unknown. Aminophylline is the ethylenediamine salt of theophylline. [See Bioavailability (F) on page 182].

Dose

Loading Dose (Aminophylline)

➥ Based upon total body weight (TBW), normal volume of distribution (Vd), a target level of 10–15 mg/L, and an assumed theophylline level of zero at the time of loading.

➥ Adults: 6–8 mg/kg aminophylline (4.8–6.4 mg/kg theophylline) administered over 30 min.

➥ Adolescents, children, and infants (12 mon–18 yr): 6–8 mg/kg aminophylline (4.8–6.4 mg/kg theophylline) administered over 30 min.

⇨ Premature newborns and patients with cystic fibrosis may have a slightly elevated Vd and require higher doses.

⇨ Some clinicians recommend 3 mg/kg aminophylline (2.4 mg/kg theophylline) in a patient who has been on therapy and that levels be drawn before administration of a loading dose. However, when previous theophylline intake is uncertain, plasma concentrations should be ascertained *before* a loading dose is administered.

Maintenance Dose

⇨ Expressed as theophylline in mg/kg/hr; based upon ideal body weight (IBW) and a target level of 10–15 mg/L, except for neonatal doses which are based upon a target level of 5–10 mg/L.

⇨ Aminophylline = theophylline/0.8. Disease and drug interactions also must be considered [see Clearance (Cl) & Half-life ($t\frac{1}{2}$) on page 185].

⇨ The following doses are expected ranges and should not be used without appropriate therapeutic drug monitoring:

- adult (non-smoker): 0.4–0.6 mg/kg/hr theophylline
- adult (smoker): 0.6–0.9 mg/kg/hr theophylline
- children (12–16 yr): 0.5–0.8 mg/kg/hr theophylline
- children (1–9 yr): 0.9–1.3 mg/kg/hr theophylline
- infants (6–52 wk): (0.008) (age in wk) + (0.21) = mg/kg/hr theophylline

       □ neonates (24–42 days): 1.5 mg/kg/Q 12 hr the-
          ophylline

       □ neonates (0–24 days): 1 mg/kg/Q 12 hr theophyl-
          line

Therapeutic & Toxic Range

Therapeutic Range

    ⇨ Asthma: 5–20 mg/L.

    ⇨ Premature neonatal apnea: 5–10 mg/L.

Toxic Concentrations

    ⇨ 13–15 mg/L: nausea, vomiting.

    ⇨ >20 mg/L: nausea, vomiting (more frequently), in-
      somnia, nervousness.

    ⇨ >40 mg/L: sinus tachycardia, atrial tachycardia, ven-
      tricular tachycardia, insomnia, nervousness.

    ⇨ >50 mg/L: seizures.

    ⇨ Do not assume toxicity will occur in stepwise fashion
      with escalating plasma concentrations. Seizures or ar-
      rhythmias can occur at lower concentrations without
      warning symptoms.

Pharmacokinetic Parameters

Bioavailability (F)

    ⇨ Oral (F = 1.0 for most products).

        □ rate of absorption can be decreased by concurrent
          administration of food or antacids

- □ enteric coated tablets should be avoided

- □ once-daily dosage forms can produce great fluctuations in plasma concentrations

- □ potentially toxic dose *dumping* has been observed when Theo-24 is administered with food

⇨ Rectal.

- □ cocoa butter-based suppositories associated with erratic absorption patterns; should not be used

- □ rectal solution and polyethylene glycol suppositories (not available commercially) are well absorbed

⇨ Intramuscular.

- □ avoid this route

- □ solution is alkaline (pH = 9.5), and injections are painful

- □ tissue pH can result in precipitation in tissue and delayed absorption

⇨ Time to peak plasma concentration (depends upon the formulation).

- □ solution and tablets: 0.5–1.0 hr

- □ sustained-release products: 3–8 hr

⇨ *Salt form (S).*

- □ aminophylline is the ethylenediamine salt of theophylline

- □ 80%–85% (contingent upon hydration) of aminophylline is available as theophylline

Table 15.1　　　　**Salt Fraction (S)**

Dosage Forms	Theophylline (%)
Uncoated Tablets,Liquid, and IV Solutions	
Aminophylline (ethylenediamine)	0.8–0.85
Elixophylline	1.0
Theophylline	1.0
Somophyllin T	1.0
Slo-Phyllin	1.0
Choledyl	0.64
Coated and Sustained Release	
Choledyl SA (oxtriphylline)	0.64
Aerolate	1.0
Slo-Phyllin Gyrocap	1.0
Somophyllin CRT	1.0
Theo-Dur	1.0
Theo-24	1.0
Theobid Dura Cap	1.0
Miscellaneous	
Dyphylline (Dihydroxypropyl theophylline)[a]	0.0
Theophylline sodium glycinate	0.45

[a]Dyphylline contains 70% theophylline by molecular weight, however, no theophylline is released *in vivo*.

Volume of Distribution (Vd)

⇨ Normal: Vd = 0.5 L/kg (0.3–0.7 L/kg).

⇨ Premature neonate: Vd = 0.7 L/kg.

⇨ Cystic fibrosis: Vd = 0.6 L/kg.

⇨ Vd should be based upon TBW if patient is not >15% above IBW.

⇨ If the patient is >15% above IBW, the practitioner may conservatively elect to calculate Vd based upon a weight between TBW and IBW.

Clearance (Cl) & Half-Life (t½). The clearance of theophylline in the adult is an average of 0.04 L/kg based upon IBW. This Cl is highly variable and is affected by numerous factors (see Table 15.2). Likewise, the t½ is highly variable (average: 8 hr) and also is affected by many factors.

Useful Pharmacokinetic Equations

Loading Dose

$$\text{Loading Dose} = \frac{(Vd)(Cp)}{(S)(F)} \qquad \text{(Eq 11, pg 19)}$$

Maintenance Dose

$$\text{Maintenance Dose} = \frac{(Cl)(Cpss\ ave)(\tau)}{(S)(F)} \qquad \text{(Eq 16, pg 28)}$$

Cl Calculated from a Steady-State Level
(IV Continuous Infusion or PO Sustained-Release (SR) Tablets.)

$$Cl = \frac{(S)(F)(Dose/\tau)}{Cpss\ ave} \qquad \text{(Eq 15, pg 26)}$$

Cl Calculated from a Nonsteady-State Level

    ⇨ *Note:* Requires iteration and an assumption of Vd (see **Basic Clinical Pharmacokinetics**, 3rd edition (pages 420–23) for more information).[1]

Table 15.2   Clearance (Cl) and Half-Life (t¹/₂)

	Cl^a (L/kg/hr)	$t^{1/2}$ (hr)	Factor[b,c,d]
Patient Group			
Nonsmoker	0.040	8–9	1.0
Smoker	0.064	5	1.6
CHF	0.016	22	0.4
Cirrhosis	0.020	17	0.5
Severe obstruction	0.031	8–10	0.8
Obesity			IBW
Children (12–16 yr)	0.05	6–7	1.25
Children (1–12 yr)	0.096	3–4	2.4
Drug Interactions			
Phenytoin	0.06	5–6	1.5
Phenobarbital	0.052	6–7	1.3
Rifampin	0.048	7	1.2
Erythromycin	0.028	12	0.7
Triacetyloleandomycin	0.028	12	0.7
Cimetidine	0.024	14	0.6
Propranolol	0.024	14	0.6

[a]The above values are means which do not reflect the dynamic nature of Cl particularly in the pediatric population.

[b]Use of clearance factors: The above stated clearance factors are utilized by multiplying the appropriate factor by the normal average clearance. For example, if a patient is a smoker, the expected patient Cl would be predicted by multiplying the patient's weight by the usual Cl (0.04 L/kg/hr) by the smoker's factor of 1.6. There is a great deal of variability in the average Cl and in the adjustment factors. In the patient who is influenced by more than one factor, (e.g., a patient who is a smoker, has severe obstructive pulmonary disease, and congestive heart failure), some clinicians would suggest that the patient's clearance be predicted as follows: $(1.6) \times (0.4) \times (0.8) \times (0.04 \text{ L/kg/hr}) \times$ patient's weight. Clearance values based on multiple adjustment factors should be used with great caution since none of the above factors have been evaluated in combination. Serum theophylline concentrations must be closely monitored. When utilizing these factors check your dosage recommendations against normal dosage recommendations to assure that they are reasonable.

[c]Predictions based on the values should not be relied upon without serum concentration monitoring.

[d]Clearance can also be decreased by influenza vaccination, BCPs, halothane, and quinolones.

Without loading dose
(nonsteady-state infusion equation)

$$Cp = \frac{(S)(F)(Dose/\tau)}{Cl}\left[1 - e^{-\left(\frac{Cl}{Vd}\right)t_{in}}\right]$$

(Pg 420)

With loading dose

$$Cp = \frac{(S)(F)(Dose/\tau)}{Cl}\left[1 - e^{-\left(\frac{Cl}{Vd}\right)t_{in}}\right] + \frac{(S)(F)(Dose/\tau)}{Vd}\left[e^{-\left(\frac{Cl}{Vd}\right)t_1}\right]$$

(Pg 420)

Serum Sampling Strategies

IV Therapy

⇨ Before administration of loading dose in patient with a history of theophylline use.

⇨ One-half hour after the end of a loading dose infusion to assess the adequacy of loading dose (not always necessary).

⇨ Levels drawn before 3–5 $t\frac{1}{2}$s after initiation of maintenance infusion should be evaluated as nonsteady-state levels. In many instances, the first level may be drawn 18–24 hr after initiation of the maintenance infusion.

⇨ Levels should be rechecked every 2–3 days after steady state has been achieved, unless the patient's clinical status warrants concern or interacting medications are added to the regimen.

Oral Therapy

⇨ **Oral liquids or nonsustained-release products:** in most instances, trough levels should be obtained just before the next dose and peak concentrations estimated.

$$\text{Cpss max} = [\text{Cpss min}] + \left[\frac{(S)(F)(\text{Dose})}{\text{Vd}} \right] \text{(Eq 15.1, pg 412)}$$

⇨ **Sustained-release (SR) products:** levels may be drawn in the period spanning the midpoint of the dosing interval to just before the next dose.

Time to Steady State. Time to steady state may be estimated by multiplying the patient's t½ by 3–5, assuming dose and interval are unchanged during that period. For example, in an adult nonsmoker, theophylline steady-state levels would be expected 24–40 hr after the initiation of the regimen.

Dialyzability

⇨ **Hemodialysis:** not significantly removed.

⇨ **Peritoneal:** not significantly removed.

⇨ **Hemoperfusion.**
  □ Significant removal
  □ Used to treat severe overdose

Monitoring Parameters

Subjective

⇨ Signs of central nervous system (CNS) stimulation.

⇨ GI/discomfort.

⇨ Dyspnea.

Objective

⇨ Serum levels.

⇨ Tremors.

⇨ Pulse.

⇨ Respiratory rate.

⇨ Breath sounds.

⇨ Arterial blood gases (ABG).

⇨ Pulmonary function tests (PFTs).

⇨ Electrocardiogram (ECG).

Drug Interactions

⇨ *Cimetidine* may inhibit the metabolism of theophylline.

⇨ *Ciprofloxacin* may inhibit the metabolism of theophylline.

⇨ *Disulfiram* may inhibit the metabolism of theophylline.

⇨ *Enoxacin* may inhibit the metabolism of theophylline.

⇨ *Erythromycin* may inhibit the metabolism of theophylline.

⇨ *Oral contraceptives* may inhibit the metabolism of theophylline.

⇨ *Phenobarbital* enhances the metabolism of theophylline.

⇨ *Phenytoin* enhances the metabolism of theophylline.

⇨ *Propranolol* may inhibit the metabolism of theophylline.

⇨ *Rifampin* enhances the metabolism of theophylline.

⇨ *Triacetyloleandomycin* may inhibit the metabolism of
theophylline.

Special Considerations

⇨ Infusion rate for IV loading dose should *not* exceed 25
mg/min.

⇨ IV compatibilities:

    □ NS

    □ ½NS

    □ ¼NS

    □ D5NS

    □ D5¼NS

    □ Lactated Ringer's

⇨ IV incompatibilities:

    □ fat emulsion

    □ many parenteral medications (it is preferable to
administer this medication from a dedicated IV
bag/bottle)

References

1. Winter ME. Basic Clinical Pharmacokinetics. 3rd ed. Vancouver: Applied Therapeutics; 1994:405–445.

2. Edwards DJ et al. In: Evans WE et al., eds. Applied Pharmacokinetics: Principles of Therapeutic Drug Monitoring. 3rd ed. Vancouver: Applied Therapeutics; 1992:13-1–13-38.

3. Erdman SM et al. An updated comparison of drug dosing methods. Part II: Theophylline. Clin Pharmacokinet. 1991;20;4:280–292.

4. Schiff GD et al. Inpatient theophylline toxicity: preventable factors. Ann Intern Med. 1991;114;9:748–753.

5. Bierman CW, Williams PV. Therapeutic monitoring of theophylline. Rationale and current status. Clin Pharmacokinet. 1989;17;6:377–384.

Notes:

Notes:

Tricyclic Antidepressants 16

(Amitriptyline, Desipramine, Imipramine, and Nortriptyline)

The tricyclic antidepressants (TCAs) represent an effective class of agents for the management of patients with depressive affective illness and various psychiatric disorders. The specific mechanism has not been fully characterized, but TCAs are believed to elicit their beneficial effect by interfering with neurotransmitter uptake and, possibly, through their anticholinergic properties.

The pharmacokinetic attributes of the TCAs have not been studied thoroughly because a variety of factors influence their disposition. Subsequently, pharmacokinetic characteristics of TCAs are loosely defined, and clinicians frequently rely upon clinical response as the primary gauge by which they adjust TCA regimens. The recent availability of practical assay procedures for therapeutic monitoring of these agents has provided an opportunity to more clearly define the pharmacokinetic characteristics of TCAs. Pharmacokinetics of the following agents are best understood: amitriptyline, desipramine, imipramine, and nortriptyline.

Dose

⇨ Dosage recommendations for the majority of TCAs range from 50–300 mg/day.

  □ nortriptyline has a lower range (30–100 mg/day)

⇨ Initial therapy should be started with a low dose and gradually increased over time.

  □ 50 mg/day in up to 4 divided doses initially

      □ increase the dose by 25–50 mg increments after ≈5 days as tolerated

      □ elderly patients typically require lower doses; up to 50% of average dose

⇨ Full antidepressant effect of TCAs is not observed for several weeks.

⇨ Once stabilized, gradually reduce to the minimally effective dose; usually given once daily (i.e., bedtime).

⇨ IM doses rarely are used but can be given.

      □ usually given in 3–4 divided doses not to exceed 100 mg/day

Therapeutic & Toxic Range

A correlation between TCA plasma concentrations and efficacy or toxicity has not been clearly established. The significant intra- and interpatient variation, presence of several active metabolites, and a variety of other factors (e.g., protein binding, variable bioavailability, wide range of Vd) that potentially can influence the pharmacokinetic parameters of TCAs, all contribute to the difficulty in defining therapeutic and toxic concentration ranges.

Therapeutic Concentrations

⇨ Vary widely (total drug levels shown):

      □ *amitriptyline:* 120–250 ng/mL (*includes metabolite*)

      □ *desipramine:* 100–250 ng/mL

      □ *imipramine:* 180–350 ng/mL (*includes metabolite*)

      □ *nortriptyline:* 50–150 ng/mL

⇨ Concentrations exceeding the therapeutic range, especially for nortriptyline, may reduce the desired therapeutic response.

⇨ Steady state usually is achieved after 1 week, but maximal therapeutic response is not seen for several weeks.

⇨ Use of free versus total drug levels has not improved the correlation between concentration, effect, and toxicity.

⇨ Clinical response rather than plasma concentrations should be used to arrive at an optimal TCA regimen.

Toxic Concentrations

⇨ Toxicity tends to occur at concentrations >500 ng/mL; concentrations >1000 ng/mL warrant withholding the TCA.

⇨ *Primary adverse events include:*

   □ anticholinergic: constipation, urinary retention, dry mouth, blurred vision, hallucinations

   □ central nervous system (CNS) effects: sedation, fatigue, tremors, seizures, extrapyramidal effects

   □ cardiovascular: orthostatic hypotension, prolonged PR, widened QRS, heart block

   □ miscellaneous: blood dyscrasias (rare), increased liver function tests (LFTs), allergy

⇨ Tolerance to most of the adverse reactions occurs with time.

⇨ Initiating therapy with a low dose which gradually is increased will minimize side effects.

Pharmacokinetic Parameters

	Bioavailability (F) average (range)	Vd (L/kg)	Protein Binding	$t^{1/2}$ (hr) average (range)
Amitriptyline	0.4 (0.3–0.6)	6.4–36	>90%	20 (10–50)
Desipramine	0.4 (0.3–0.5)	15–60	70%–90%	20 (7–60)
Imipramine	0.4 (0.2–0.7)	9.3–23	70%–96%	20 (8–20)
Nortriptyline	0.5 (0.45–0.7)	14–38	>90%	30 (16–90)

Bioavailability (F)

⇨ TCAs primarily are available as oral formulations (except amitriptyline and imipramine):

□ *amitriptyline:*

○ tablets: 10, 25, 50, 75, 100, and 150 mg

○ injectable: 10 mg/mL

□ *desipramine:*

○ tablets: 10, 25, 50, 75, 100, and 150 mg

○ capsules: 25 and 50 mg

□ *imipramine:*

○ tablets: 10, 25, and 50 mg

○ capsules: 75, 100, 125, and 150 mg

○ injectable: 12.5 mg/mL

□ *nortriptyline:*

○ capsules: 10, 25, 50, and 75 mg

○ solution: 10 mg/5 mL

⇨ IM injections rarely are used.

    □ higher parent to metabolite ratio relative to oral formulations, due to less influence from first-pass effect

⇨ Bioavailability of all TCAs averages 0.4, but varies widely due to first-pass effect (F = 30%–70%) (see Table).

⇨ Oral TCAs are well absorbed in the GI tract with peak plasma concentrations occurring in 2–8 hr.

    □ peak concentration varies substantially with TCAs

    □ differences in absorption may exist between different brands (i.e., generic versus brand)

Clearance (Cl) & Half-Life (t½)

⇨ Primary route of elimination is through the liver to several active metabolites.

    □ amitriptyline is metabolized to nortriptyline

    □ imipramine is metabolized to desipramine

⇨ Consider active metabolites when monitoring TCA plasma concentrations.

⇨ Minimal amounts (i.e., <5%) of parent TCAs are excreted unchanged in the urine.

    □ a greater percentage of metabolites are renally excreted

⇨ Cl of TCAs will vary significantly from patient to patient.

    □ average values: 10 mL/kg/min (0.6 L/kg/hr)

    □ a genetic predisposition associated with the Cl of TCAs may exist

⇨ Patients with impaired liver function will have reduced Cl which may require dosage adjustment.

⇨ Several drugs may influence the Cl of TCAs. (See Drug Interactions.)

⇨ t½ for each TCA varies considerably but averages 20 hr (see Table).

Volume of Distribution (Vd)

⇨ Highly lipophilic drugs with extensive tissue and protein distribution.

  □ present in cardiac tissue, CNS, lungs, liver, and breast milk

  □ despite lipid solubility, very little distribution into adipose tissue

⇨ Vd varies considerably; most values are in the range of 15–20 L/kg.

⇨ Highly bound to plasma and tissue proteins (free fraction is 5%–10%).

  □ factors that influence protein (mostly α-1-acid glycoprotein) likely will influence Vd and plasma concentration of TCAs (see **Basic Clinical Pharmacokinetics**, 3rd edition for more information).[3]

Serum Sampling Strategies

⇨ Routine serum levels usually are not advocated due to their poor correlation with effect or toxicity.

⇨ Clinical response is a more useful gauge for efficacy or toxicity.

⇨ Serum levels may be beneficial in the following situations:

- patients who do not respond despite an adequate dose and appropriate duration of therapy
- patients at risk for toxicity (i.e., the elderly or patients with decreased hepatic function)
- patients in which compliance is questioned

⇨ It is best to obtain plasma concentrations after steady state is achieved ($\approx$1 wk).

⇨ The long $t\frac{1}{2}$ suggests the timing of the sample collection is not critical.

- peak levels are hard to determine and troughs tend to occur at bedtime in patients on a QD regimen; it is best to obtain the TCA concentration in the middle of a dosing interval (12 hr)

Dialyzability

Hemodialysis & Peritoneal

⇨ TCAs are not significantly influenced by either hemodialysis or peritoneal dialysis. The drug may be removed from the serum; however, the majority of the drug in the body is extensively bound to tissue and protein. Therefore, dialysis has little impact on the total body stores of TCA.

Monitoring Parameters

Subjective

⇨ Improvement in depressive behavior.

⇨ Complaints of anticholinergic effects (e.g., dry mouth and blurred vision).

Objective

⇨ Vital signs (orthostatic hypotension).

⇨ Electrocardiogram (ECG) (if toxicity is suspected).

⇨ TCA plasma concentrations (if necessary).

Drug Interactions

⇨ *Adrenergic agents.* The effects of norepinephrine, epinephrine, isoproterenol, phenylephrine, and other direct acting sympathomimetics may be greatly enhanced when administered concurrently with TCAs.

⇨ *Alcohol.* Acute ingestion of alcohol may competitively inhibit the metabolism of TCAs and result in elevations of TCA plasma concentrations. Conversely, chronic alcohol ingestion is more likely to induce hepatic metabolism and accelerate the elimination of TCAs.

⇨ *Anticholinergic agents* may have an additive effect when administered concurrently with TCAs.

⇨ *Anticonvulsants (carbamazepine, phenytoin, barbiturates)* may enhance the Cl of TCAs.

⇨ *Cigarette smoking* may induce hepatic metabolism of TCAs resulting in an enhanced Cl of the antidepressants.

⇨ *Cimetidine.* Elevation in TCA plasma concentrations secondary to competitive inhibition of hepatic enzymes may be observed when cimetidine is administered concurrently.

⇨ *Clonidine.* TCAs may interfere with the uptake of clonidine resulting in diminished antihypertensive effects of clonidine.

⇨ *Fluoxetine* may inhibit the metabolism of TCAs and elevate TCA plasma concentrations.

⇨ *Guanethidine.* TCAs may interfere with the uptake of guanethidine resulting in diminished antihypertensive effects of guanethidine.

⇨ *Haloperidol* may inhibit the metabolism of TCAs and elevate TCA plasma concentrations.

⇨ *Monoamine oxidase inhibitors (MAOIs).* Administration of TCAs with MAOIs may result in a hyperpyrexia, hypertension, confusion, and seizures.

⇨ *Sedatives* may have an additive effect when administered concurrently with TCAs.

Special Considerations

⇨ Due to their anticholinergic effects, TCAs should be used with caution in patients with prostatic hypertrophy, urinary retention, or narrow-angle glaucoma.

⇨ Avoid abrupt withdrawal of TCAs, especially in patients receiving chronic antidepressant therapy.

⇨ Elderly patients and those with underlying heart disease at risk for toxicity and should be monitored closely when TCA therapy is initiated.

⤳ *Overdose of TCAs.*

- ❑ acute toxicity due to TCA overdose usually is associated with:

    - ○ CNS effects which may progress to seizures, respiratory depression, and coma

    - ○ cardiac problems including cardiac arrest, congestive heart failure (CHF), and slowed conduction arrhythmias

    - ○ acidosis and electrolyte imbalances

- ❑ management consists of:

    - ○ supportive care and correction of any acid/base and electrolyte abnormalities

    - ○ continuous electrocardiogram (ECG) monitoring

    - ○ gastric lavage to empty the stomach

    - ○ avoid inducing emesis due to the possibility of a rapid decrease in mentation and possible aspiration

    - ○ administration of activated charcoal to reduce absorption

    - ○ dialysis is not effective because of extensive binding to tissues and proteins

References

1. DeVane CL, Jarecke CR. Cyclic antidepressants. In: Evans WE et al., eds. Applied Pharmacokinetics: Principles of Therapeutic Drug Monitoring. 3rd ed. Vancouver: Applied Therapeutics; 1992:33-1–33-47.

2. Wells BG. Tricyclic antidepressants. In: Taylor WT, Diers-Cav-iness MH, eds. A Textbook for Clinical Application of Thera-peutic Drug Monitoring. Irving: Abbott Laboratories Diagnos-tic Division; 1986:449–465.

3. Winter ME. Basic Clinical Pharmacokinetics. 3rd ed. Vancou-ver: Applied Therapeutics; 1994.

Notes:

Valproic Acid   17

Valproic acid (n-dipropylacetic acid), a broad spectrum antiepileptic drug, is used to treat myoclonic, absence, and co-existing absence and tonic-clonic seizures. Valproic acid also is used to treat bipolar affective disorders refractory to lithium or other agents.

While the precise mechanism of action of valproic acid is not known, it may elicit its action by increasing central nervous system (CNS) concentrations of the inhibitory neurotransmitter γ-aminobutyric acid (GABA) or by enhancing the post-receptor effect of GABA. Valproic acid is interesting from a pharmacokinetic standpoint for several reasons: it affects the pharmacokinetics of several medications; in the therapeutic range, its concentration is sufficient to saturate protein binding sites; and it is associated with several concentration-related side effects.

Dose

Loading Dose

- ⇨ Adults and adolescents (monotherapy):
  5–15 mg/kg/day.

- ⇨ Adults and adolescents (polytherapy):
  10–30 mg/kg/day.

- ⇨ Children (1–12 yr)(monotherapy): 15 mg/kg/day.

- ⇨ Children (1–12 yr)(polytherapy): 15–30 mg/kg/day.

- ⇨ *Note:* doses generally are increased at weekly intervals by 5–10 mg/kg/day.

Maintenance Dose

⇨ Adults and adolescents (monotherapy): up to 60 mg/kg/day.

⇨ Adults and adolescents (polytherapy): up to 60 mg/kg/day.

⇨ Children(1–12 yr) (monotherapy): up to 100 mg/kg/day.

⇨ Children (1–12 yr) (polytherapy): up to 100 mg/kg/day.

⇨ *Note:* FDA approved only up to 60 mg/kg/day.

Therapeutic & Toxic Ranges

Therapeutic Range

⇨ 50–100 mg/L.

Toxic Levels

⇨ Plasma concentrations >100 mg/L are not necessarily associated with signs and symptoms of toxicity.

⇨ **Side effects**

  ◻ gastrointestinal disturbances are reported frequently and are usually dose related

    ○ pancreatitis

    ○ anorexia

    ○ weight gain

    ○ nausea

    ○ vomiting

- □ neurological
    - ○ drowsiness
    - ○ paresthesias
    - ○ mental or behavioral changes
- □ hematological
- □ thrombocytopenia (dose related)
    - ○ neutropenia
    - ○ bone marrow suppression
- □ dermatologic
    - ○ rash
    - ○ alopecia
- □ hepatotoxicity
    - ○ acute hepatotoxicity: death has been reported in several cases; usually presents within six months of initiation of therapy; more common in children treated with multiple anticonvulsants
    - ○ asymptomatic enzyme elevation

Pharmacokinetic Parameters

Bioavailability (F)

⇨ Absorption complete (F = 1.0).

⇨ *Time to peak concentration:*
- □ enteric coated tablets: 2–6 hr
- □ capsules: 1–3 hr
- □ syrup: 0.5–1 hr
- □ *note:* time to peak may increase if the medication is administered with food

⇨ Salt fraction (S) = 1.0.

  □ quantities of valproic acid are labeled on both valproic acid and divalproex sodium products

Volume of Distribution (Vd)

⇨ Vd = 0.14 L/kg (0.1–0.5 L/kg).

⇨ Vd is affected by alterations in serum albumin, renal failure, and capacity-limited binding at concentrations >50 mg/L.

Clearance (Cl) & Half-Life (t½)

⇨ Clearance (Cl).

  □ adults: 8 mL/kg/hr (6–10 mL/kg/hr)

  □ children: 13 mL/kg/hr

  □ *note:* Cl may be greater in patients being treated with multiple antiepileptic drugs

⇨ Half-life (t½).

  □ adults: 10–12 hr

  □ children: 6–8 hr

Useful Pharmacokinetic Equations

Dose

$$\text{Dose} = \frac{(\text{Cpss min})(\text{Vd})(1 - e^{-Kd\tau})}{(S)(F)(e^{-Kd\tau})} \qquad \text{(Eq 18.3, pg 469)}$$

Cpss max

$$\text{Cpss max} = [\text{Cpss min}] + \left[\frac{(S)(F)(\text{Dose})}{\text{Vd}} \right] \qquad \text{(Eq 15.1, pg 412)}$$

Cpss min

$$\text{Cpss min} = \frac{\dfrac{(S)(F)(Dose)}{Vd}}{(1 - e^{-Kd\tau})} (e^{-Kd\tau})$$

(Eq 47, pg 55)

Serum Sampling Strategies

⇨ Trough concentrations usually are monitored because of problems associated with peak concentrations (e.g., capacity-limited protein binding, variability in time-to-peak).

⇨ Peak concentrations can be estimated from known trough values.

⇨ Steady-state concentrations usually are achieved 2–3 days following initiation of medication or dose changes.

⇨ Serum samples should be taken 2–3 days following:

  ▫ initiation of medication

  ▫ dose or interval changes

  ▫ addition or discontinuation of other medications which enhance or inhibit the metabolism of valproic acid

⇨ Plasma concentrations should be measured immediately if there is an alteration in seizure activity.

Dialyzability

⇨ Hemodialysis: not removed.

Monitoring Parameters

Subjective

⇨ Drowsiness.

⇨ Lethargy.

⇨ GI discomfort.

Objective

⇨ Seizure activity.

⇨ Complete blood count (CBC).

⇨ Liver function tests (LFTs).

⇨ Renal function.

Drug Interactions

⇨ *Carbamazepine* may reduce valproic acid levels.

⇨ *Clonazepam*. When used with valproic acid, the combination may precipitate absence seizures.

⇨ *Phenobarbital*. Phenobarbital Cl may be reduced by as much as 40% in patients being treated with valproic acid. Phenobarbital may reduce valproic acid levels.

⇨ *Phenytoin*. Valproic acid will displace phenytoin from protein binding sites, reducing total plasma concentrations but not affecting the unbound concentration. Phenytoin may reduce valproic acid levels.

References

1. Winter ME. Basic Clinical Pharmacokinetics. 3rd ed. Vancouver: Applied Therapeutics; 1994:463–473.

2. Levy RH et al. Carbamazepine, Valproic Acid, Phenobarbital, and Ethosuximide. In: Evans WE et al., eds. Applied Pharmacokinetics: Principles of Therapeutic Drug Monitoring. 3rd ed. Vancouver: Applied Therapeutics; 1992:26-1–26-29.

3. Choonara IA, Rane A. Therapeutic Monitoring of Anticonvulsants, state of the art. Clin Pharmacokinet. 1990;18(4):318–328.

Notes:

Vancomycin   18

Vancomycin has had an impressive record for more than 30 years because of its excellent activity against gram-positive organisms (especially methicillin-resistant staphylococci) and lack of resistance problems. The antibiotic has multiple mechanisms of action and this may be the reason for its success. Vancomycin is believed to cause a bactericidal effect by inhibiting bacterial cell wall synthesis, altering the permeability of cytoplasmic membranes, and inhibiting RNA synthesis.

Vancomycin is well tolerated. Many of its side effects have been attributed to impurities present in earlier preparations, and "red man syndrome" has been related to the rate of administration. Current preparations administered over an appropriate duration are associated with few adverse reactions.

No other approved antibiotics are reasonable alternatives to vancomycin. The investigational agent, teicoplanin, is a related compound; however, clinical trials have not demonstrated any significant advantages over vancomycin.

Dose

Vancomycin should be administered by intermittent IV infusion over at least 30–60 min and the dose should be based upon the patient's ideal body weight (IBW), renal function, and severity of infection. In the majority of cases, the daily dose should not exceed 2 gm/day.

Loading Dose

⇨ Based upon an estimate of the patient's Vd and the desired plasma concentration.

⇨ General guidelines for loading doses vary significantly (range: 8–25 mg/kg).

Maintenance Dose and Interval

⇨ Frequently determined by vancomycin Cl and desired peak and trough levels.

⇨ Cl_{Cr} is used to calculate vancomycin Cl.

⇨ Dosage interval must take into account patient's renal function.

Dosing Nomograms

⇨ Developed to assist in determining appropriate vancomycin regimens.

⇨ Useful as initial guidelines until patient-specific data are available to "fine-tune" the dosage regimen.

⇨ Several of these nomograms are listed below with brief descriptions and comments.

- □ Lake method (see Figure 18.1)
  - ○ simple and fairly accurate
  - ○ dose based upon a corrected weight; usually can use IBW (except in obese individuals)
  - ○ interval based upon various Cl_{Cr}
  - ○ no loading dose used
- □ Matzke method (see Figure 18.2)
  - ○ separate loading and maintenance doses
  - ○ loading dose = 25 mg/kg
  - ○ maintenance dose = 19 mg/kg
  - ○ dosage interval is read off the nomogram (Cl_{Cr})

- based upon one-compartment model
- produces aggressive concentrations
- useful in patients with poor renal function; tends to overestimate dose in patients with normal renal function

□ Moellering method (see Figure 18.3)

- determine daily dose from nomogram
- calculate Cl_{Cr} in mL/kg/min
- interval is arbitrarily determined
- based upon a three-compartment model
- designed to produce a Cpss of 15 mg/L

□ Nielsen method

$$\text{Daily Maintenance Dose} \atop \text{(mg/day)} = (15)(Cl_{Cr} \text{ in mL/min}) + 150$$

- interval is arbitrarily determined
- based upon producing a desired Cpss of 20 mg/L

Therapeutic & Toxic Ranges

The therapeutic peak and trough concentrations for vancomycin are more loosely defined than those described for aminoglycosides. Correlations between plasma concentrations and efficacy and toxicity have not been clearly established. Reported peak plasma concentrations range from 15–40 mg/L and trough concentrations from 5–15 mg/L. The wide range in plasma concentrations has been attributed to sample timing (see Serum Sampling Strategies on page 221).

Calculated Dose = 8 mg/kg CBW

Equation 1. Lean body weight (LBW)

LBW for males = 50 kg + 2.3(height − 60 in)

LBW for females = 45.5 kg + 2.3(height − 60 in)

Equation 2. Corrected body weight (CBW)

CBW = [(TBW − LBW)(0.4)] + LBW

Dose Interval

Equation 3.

$$\frac{Cl_{Cr} \text{ for males}}{\text{(mL/min)}} = \frac{(140 - \text{age})(\text{wt in kg})}{(72)(\text{SrCr})}$$

$$\frac{Cl_{Cr} \text{ for females}}{\text{(mL/min)}} = (0.85)\frac{(140 - \text{age})(\text{wt in kg})}{(72)(\text{SrCr})}$$

Estimated Cl_{Cr} (mL/min)	Dosing Interval (hr)
≥90	6
70–89	8
45–69	12
30–44	18
15–29	24

Note: If SrCr is <1.0, a value of 1.0 should be substituted

Figure 18.1. Lake Method. Simplified method for initiating vancomycin therapy. Reprinted with permission from reference 4.

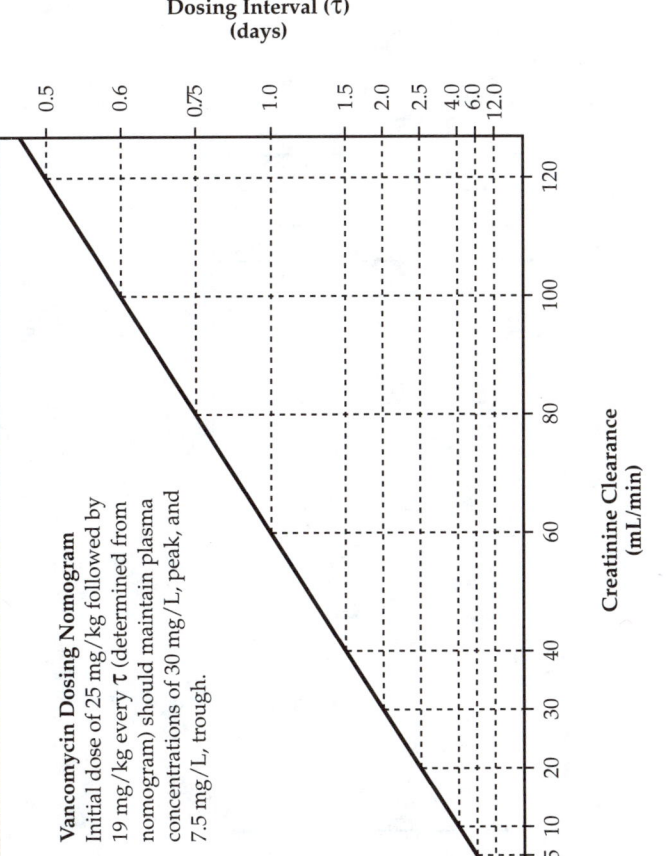

Dosing Interval (τ)
(days)

Vancomycin Dosing Nomogram
Initial dose of 25 mg/kg followed by
19 mg/kg every τ (determined from
nomogram) should maintain plasma
concentrations of 30 mg/L, peak, and
7.5 mg/L, trough.

Creatinine Clearance
(mL/min)

Figure 18.2. Matzke nomogram for dosing vancomycin in patients with various
degrees of renal function. Reprinted with permission from reference 3.

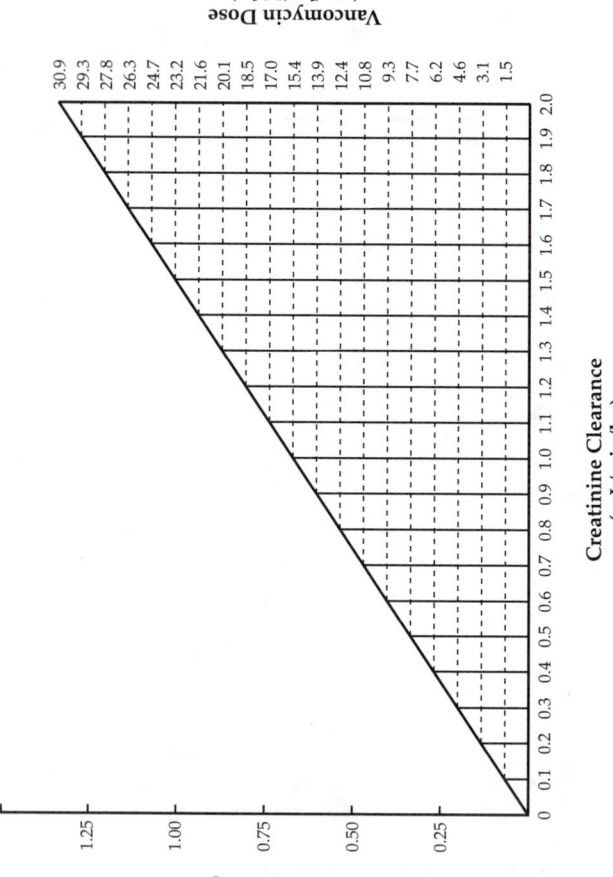

Figure 18.3. Moellering nomogram for dosing vancomycin in patients with various degrees of renal function. Reprinted with permission from reference 6.

Toxicity

⇨ **Primary toxic effects:**
- □ nephrotoxicity
- □ ototoxicity
- □ red man syndrome
- □ phlebitis
- □ neutropenia
- □ drug fever

⇨ Poor correlation between plasma concentrations and related toxicities.

⇨ Ototoxicity appears to occur when concentrations exceed 80 mg/L.

⇨ Nephrotoxicity is rare and most likely occurs with concomitant administration of aminoglycosides (see Drug Interactions on page 223).

⇨ Administration rate-related adverse reactions (i.e., Red Man syndrome) often can be avoided by slowing administration rate.

Pharmacokinetic Parameters

Bioavailability (F)

⇨ Both oral and parenteral formulations of vancomycin are available.

⇨ Oral absorption is very poor (i.e., <5%) and only is used to treat pseudomembranous colitis and staphylococcal enteritis.

⇨ Intrathecal and intraventricular administration may be needed for central nervous system (CNS) infections.

⇨ IM injections should be avoided due to local irritation.

Volume of Distribution (Vd)

⇨ Widely distributed with 50% bound to protein (albumin).

⇨ Vd = 0.7 L/kg (range: 0.5 to 1.0 L/kg).

⇨ Penetrates into cerebrospinal fluid (CSF) in the presence of inflamed meninges.

⇨ Initial distribution phase (α phase) is present and varies from 30–120 min; large changes in concentration occur with small time changes during the distribution phase.

Clearance (Cl) & Half-Life (t½)

⇨ 80%–90% excreted renally via glomerular filtration.

⇨ Metabolism accounts for a slight (i.e., 5%) portion of elimination.

⇨ Cl_{Cr} can be used to estimate vancomycin Cl.

   ▫ vancomycin Cl = 0.65 (Cl_{Cr}) (Total Body Weight)
   ▫ *Note:* this method does not work well in neonates or pediatric patients

⇨ Decreased Cl in the elderly and in patients with decreased renal function.

⇨ t½ = 6–8 hr; may be prolonged to 7 days in severe renal impairment.

Useful Pharmacokinetic Equations

Estimating Initial Pharmacokinetic Parameters:

Volume of distribution (L)

$$Vd = 0.7 \text{ L/kg (Based upon actual body weight)}$$

Vancomycin clearance (L/hr)

⇨ Use Cl_{Cr} to calculate vancomycin Cl:

$$\begin{array}{c} Cl_{Cr} \text{ for Males} \\ \text{(mL/min)} \end{array} = \frac{(140 - \text{Age})(\text{Weight})}{(72)(\text{SrCr}_{ss})} \qquad \text{(Eq 63, pg 95)}$$

$$Cl_{Cr} \text{ for Females} = (0.85) \frac{(140 - \text{Age})(\text{Weight})}{(72)(\text{SrCr}_{ss})} \qquad \text{(Eq 64, pg 95)}$$

$$\text{Vancomycin Cl} = (0.65)(Cl_{Cr} \text{ in mL/kg/min})\left(\begin{array}{c} \text{Total Body} \\ \text{Weight in kg} \end{array}\right)$$
$$\text{(Eq 18.1, pg 476)}$$

⇨ Convert units from mL/min to L/hr:

$$\begin{array}{c} Cl_{van} \\ \text{(L/hr)} \end{array} = \left(\begin{array}{c} Cl_{van} \\ \text{in mL/min} \end{array}\right)\left(\frac{1 \text{ L}}{1000 \text{ mL}}\right)\left(\frac{60 \text{ min}}{1 \text{ hr}}\right)$$

⇨ Elimination rate constant (hr^{-1}) and $t\frac{1}{2}$ (hr).

$$\begin{array}{c} Kd \\ (hr^{-1}) \end{array} = \frac{Cl \text{ (in L/hr)}}{Vd \text{ (in L)}} \qquad \text{(Eq 27, pg 41)}$$

$$\begin{array}{c} t\frac{1}{2} \\ \text{(hr)} \end{array} = \frac{(0.693)(Vd)}{Cl} \qquad \text{(Eq 32, pg 43)}$$

Determining an Initial Dosage Regimen:

Loading dose (mg)

$$\text{Loading Dose} = \frac{(Vd)(Cp \text{ desired})}{(S)(F)}$$

(Eq 11, pg 19)

Maintenance dose (mg)

$$\text{Maintenance Dose} = \frac{(Cl)(Cpss \text{ ave})(\tau)}{(S)(F)}$$

(Eq 16, pg 28)

⇨ The estimated t½ should be considered when choosing a dosage interval.

Maintenance Dose (mg)
Based Upon a Desired Cpss max and Cpss min:

$$\text{Dose} = \frac{(Vd)(Cpss \text{ max} - Cpss \text{ min})}{(S)(F)}$$

(Eq 18.2, pg 483)

Expected Cpss max and
Cpss min for a Given Dosage Regimen:

$$\text{Cpss max} = \frac{\dfrac{(S)(F)(Dose)}{Vd}}{(1 - e^{-Kd\tau})}$$

(Eq 43, pg 53)

$$\text{Cpss min} = \frac{\dfrac{(S)(F)(Dose)}{Vd}}{(1 - e^{-Kd\tau})} (e^{-Kd\tau})$$

(Eq 47, pg 55)

Serum Sampling Strategies

⮕ In most situations, peak and trough studies are used to evaluate vancomycin dosage regimens. Follow-up evaluations are conducted at various intervals depending upon the clinical situation or changing factors that may influence the pharmacokinetic parameters of vancomycin. However, vancomycin plasma concentrations obtained on the first dose are of limited value.

⮕ A large degree of confusion surrounds the questions of when to draw vancomycin concentrations (particularly peaks) and what should be the optimal concentrations. The source of the controversy is vancomycin's bi-exponential decay. There are three common approaches to obtaining vancomycin plasma concentrations:

   ☐ 1) Peak concentrations should be obtained ≈1–3 hr after the end of the infusion to avoid the sharply declining distribution (α) phase.

   ☐ 2) Peak concentrations should be obtained just after the end of the vancomycin infusion to determine the maximal (peak) concentration.

   ☐ 3) Peak concentrations should not be used; instead, obtain a trough concentration just before a subsequent dose. If the trough is within an acceptable range, the peak concentration also must be acceptable.

⮕ Since the minimum inhibitory concentration (MIC) of vancomycin against most staphylococci rarely exceeds 1–2 mg/L, *maintaining* a trough between 5–10 mg/L is clinically acceptable and does not put the patient in toxic Cp ranges.

⮕ Interpretation of the plasma concentration is critical. A peak concentration of 16 mg/L may be appropriate if the concentration was obtained 2 hr after the end of the infusion; however, the same may not be true if the concentration has been drawn at the end of the infusion (i.e., it may be too low).

Dialyzability

Hemodialysis

⇨ Vancomycin is not significantly removed by hemodialysis.

⇨ Supplemental doses are not required.

Peritoneal

⇨ Vancomycin is not significantly removed by peritoneal dialysis.

⇨ Supplemental doses are not required.

Monitoring Parameters

Subjective

⇨ Phlebitis.

⇨ Rash, flushing (histamine release).

Objective

⇨ Vancomycin plasma concentrations.

⇨ Microbiology cultures.

⇨ White blood cell (WBC) count and differential.

⇨ Temperature (afebrile).

⇨ Vital signs.

⇨ BUN/SrCr.

⇨ Urinary output (I/O).

⇨ Audiometry testing (only in high risk patients).

Drug Interactions

Aminoglycosides

⇨ The incidence of vancomycin nephrotoxicity is greatly enhanced with concurrent aminoglycoside administration.

⇨ Reports have suggested a <5% prevalence of nephrotoxicity with vancomycin alone; however, it has been as high as 35% in patients receiving both vancomycin and an aminoglycoside.

Special Considerations

Rate of Infusion

⇨ Infuse vancomycin doses over at least 30–60 min.

⇨ If flushing, rash, hypotension, or tachycardia develop (i.e., Red Man syndrome), temporarily discontinue the infusion, medicate with antihistamines, and resume the infusion at a slower rate after symptoms resolve.

Dosing in Obese Patients

⇨ Use of an adjusted dosing weight in patients with significant obesity has been suggested to account for that portion of the dose (i.e., 40%) distributed into adipose tissue: [(0.4) (actual body weight − IBW) + IBW].

References

1. Winter ME. Basic Clinical Pharmacokinetics. 3rd ed. Vancouver: Applied Therapeutics; 1994:474–499.

2. Matzke GR. Vancomycin. In: Evans WE et al., eds. Applied Pharmacokinetics: Principles of Therapeutic Drug Monitoring. 3rd ed. Vancouver: Applied Therapeutics; 1992:15-1–15-31.

3. Matzke GR et al. Pharmacokinetics of vancomycin in patients with various degrees of renal function. Antimicrob Agents Chemother. 1984;25:433–437.

4. Lake KD, Peterson CD. Evaluation of a method for initiating vancomycin therapy: experience in 205 patients. Pharmacotherapy. 1988;8(5):284–286.

5. Rybak MJ, Boike SC. Monitoring vancomycin therapy. Drug Intell Clin Pharm. 1986;20:757–761.

6. Moellering RC et al. Vancomycin therapy in patients with impaired renal function: a nomogram for dosing. Ann Intern Med. 1981;94:343–346.

7. Nielsen HE et al. Renal excretion of vancomycin in renal disease. Acta Med Scand. 1975;197:261–264.

Notes:

Appendix I

Nomogram for Calculating the Body Surface Area of Children[a]

Height	Surface Area	Weight

(Height scale: cm 120 / 47 in down to cm 25 / 10 in)

(Surface Area scale: 1.10 m² down to 0.074 m²)

(Weight scale: kg 40.0 / 90 lb down to kg 1.0 / 2.2 lb)

[a] From the formula of DuBois and DuBois. Arch Intern Med. 1916;17:863: $S = W^{0.425} \times H^{0.725} \times 71.84$, or $\log S = 0.425 \log W + 0.725 \log H + 1.8564$, where S = Body surface area in cm², W = Weight in kg, H = Height in cm.

Nomogram for Calculating the Body Surface Area of Adults[a]

Height	Surface Area	Weight

[a] From the formula of DuBois and DuBois. Arch Intern Med. 1916;17:863: $S = W^{0.425} \times H^{0.725} \times 71.84$, or $\log S = 0.425 \log W + 0.725 \log H + 1.8564$, where S = Body surface area in cm^2, W = Weight in kg, H = Height in cm. Reprinted with permission from the publisher. Lontmer C., ed. Geigy Scientific Tables. 8th edition. Volume 1: Basle: Ciba-Geigy. 1981:226-27.

Appendix II:

Glossary of Terms and Abbreviations

Ab: See Amount of Drug in the Body.

Accumulation Factor: $1/1 - e^{-Kd\tau}$ or the degree to which a maintenance dose will accumulate when steady state is achieved.

Adjusted Body Weight: A weight for dosing drugs in obese patients which is between ideal body weight and total body weight.

Administration Rate (R_A): The average rate at which a drug is administered to the patient.

Alpha (α): a) Fraction of the total plasma concentration which is free or unbound. b) The initial half-life in a two compartment model, usually representing distribution.

Amount of Drug in the Body (Ab): The total amount of active drug which is in the body at any given time.

Average Steady-State Concentration (Cpss ave): The average plasma drug concentration at steady state.

Beta (β): a) Second decay half-life in a two compartment model, usually representing elimination. b) The fraction of total plasma concentration which is bound to plasma proteins.

Bioavailability (F): The fraction of an administered dose which reaches the systemic circulation.

Body Surface Area (BSA): The surface area of a patient, as determined by weight and height (see Appendix I).

Bolus Dose: A model for rapid input of a dose into the body or an individual dose usually given by intravenous injection.

BSA: See Body Surface Area.

CAPD: See Continuous Ambulatory Peritoneal Dialysis.

Cl: See Clearance.

$Cl_{adjusted}$: Clearance of a patient which has been adjusted or altered for the presence of a disease state such as renal failure or heart failure.

Cl_{CAPD}: Drug clearance by peritoneal dialysis.

Cl_{Cr}: See Creatinine Clearance.

Cl_{dial}: Drug clearance by dialysis.

Cl_m: See Clearance, metabolic.

Cl_{pat}: Drug clearance of patient, usually associated with decreased renal function.

Cl_r: See Clearance, renal.

Clearance (Cl_t or Cl): Total body clearance is a measure of how well a patient can metabolize or eliminate drugs. It is used to calculate maintenance doses or average steady-state plasma concentrations.

Clearance, metabolic (Cl_m): A measure of how well the body can metabolize drugs. The major metabolic organ is usually the liver.

Clearance, renal (Cl_r): A measure of how well the kidneys can excrete unchanged or unmetabolized drugs. It is usually assumed to be proportional to creatinine clearance.

Cp: See Plasma Concentration.

Cp′: Plasma concentration measured in patients with altered plasma protein binding.

Cp^0: The initial plasma concentration at the beginning of a decay phase, usually following a loading dose.

ΔCp: Change in plasma concentration resulting from a single dose.

Cp desired: Plasma concentration desired following an incremental loading dose.

Cp free: Unbound or free plasma concentration.

$Cp_{NormalBinding}$: Plasma concentration that would be observed or measured if patient's plasma protein binding is normal.

$Cp_{initial}$: Plasma concentration present in patient before incremental loading dose.

$\textbf{Cp}_{t_{in}}$: Plasma concentration at the end of a short infusion or at the end of absorption.

Cpss ave: Average plasma concentration at steady state.

Cpss max: The maximum or peak concentration at steady state, when a constant dose is administered at a constant dosing interval.

Cpss min: The minimum or trough concentration at steady state, when a constant dose is administered at a constant dosing interval.

Creatinine Clearance (Cl_{Cr}): A measure of the kidney's ability to eliminate creatinine from the body. Total renal function is usually assumed to be proportional to creatinine clearance.

Dosing Interval (τ): The time interval between doses when a drug is given intermittently.

Dry Weight: Weight of patient before excessive fluid gain.

Dwell Time (T_D): The time between instillation and removal of a peritoneal dialysis exchange volume.

$\textbf{e}^{-\textbf{Kdt}}$: Fraction remaining at the end of a time interval.

$\textbf{1- e}^{-\textbf{Kdt}}$: a) Fraction lost during a dosing interval at steady state, if $t = \tau$. b) Fraction of steady state achieved during a constant infusion "t" hours after starting the infusion.

Elimination Rate Constant (Kd): The fractional rate of drug loss from the body or the fraction of the volume of distribution which is cleared of drug during a time interval.

Elimination Rate (R_E): The amount of drug eliminated from the body during a time interval.

Extraction Ratio: Fraction of drug which is removed from the blood or plasma as it passes through the eliminating organ.

F: See Bioavailability.

First-Pass: Drug removed from the blood or plasma, following absorption from the gastrointestinal tract, before reaching the systemic circulation.

First-Order Elimination: A process whereby the amount or concentration of drug in the body diminishes logarithmically over time. The rate of elimination is proportional to the drug concentration.

Half-Life (t½): Time required for the plasma concentration to be reduced to one-half of the original value.

Half-Life, alpha (αt½): Initial decay half-life usually representing distribution of drug into the tissue or slowly equilibrating second compartment in a two-compartment model.

Half-life, beta (βt½): Second decay half-life; usually represents the elimination half-life. Half-life, beta for most drugs can be calculated using the elimination rate constant.

IBW: See Ideal Body Weight.

Ideal Body Weight: Body weight used as an estimate of non-obese weight.

Incremental Loading Dose: An adjusted loading dose required to achieve a desired plasma concentration (Cp desired) when a pre-existing plasma concentration (Cp observed) is present.

Initial Volume of Distribution (Vi): Initial volume into which the drug rapidly equilibrates following an intravenous bolus injection.

Iterative Search: A trial and error process to determine patient-specific pharmacokinetic parameters when direct solutions are not possible due to the nature of the pharmacokinetic model being resolved.

Kd: See Elimination Rate Constant.

$Kd_{adjusted}$: Elimination rate constant which has been adjusted or altered for the presence of a disease state such as renal failure.

Kd_{dial}: Elimination rate constant representing both the patient's drug clearance and the drug clearance by dialysis.

Km (Michaelis-Menton Constant): Plasma concentration at which the rate of metabolism is occurring at half the maximum rate.

$K_{metabolic}$ (K_m): The elimination rate constant calculated from the metabolic clearance and the volume of distribution (Cl_m/Vd).

K_{renal} (K_r): The elimination rate constant calculated from the renal clearance and the volume of distribution (Cl_r/Vd).

Linear Pharmacokinetics: Assumes the elimination rate constant is not affected by plasma drug concentration and that the rate of drug elimination is directly proportional to the concentration of drug in plasma.

ln: Natural logarithm using the base 2.718 rather than 10 which is used for the common logarithm or log.

Loading Dose: Initial total dose required to rapidly achieve a desired plasma concentration.

Maintenance Dose: The dose required to replace the amount of drug lost from the body so that a desired plasma concentration can be maintained.

Mass Balance: The process of comparing drug administration rate (R_A) to the rate of change of drug in the body [$(\Delta Cp)(Vd/t)$] in order to estimate drug elimination rate (R_E).

(N): The number of doses that have been administered at a fixed-dosing interval.

One-Compartment Model: Assumes that drug distributes equally to all areas of the body. Most drugs can be modeled this way if sampling during the initial distribution phase is avoided.

P_{NL} or P': Plasma protein concentration. P_{NL} refers to the normal plasma protein concentration and P' refers to the plasma protein concentration of the specific patient.

Pharmacokinetics: Study of the absorption, distribution, metabolism, and excretion of a drug and its metabolites in the body.

Plasma Concentration (Cp): Concentration of drug in plasma. Usually refers to the total drug concentration and includes both the bound and free drug.

R_A: See Administration Rate.

R_E: See Elimination Rate.

S: See Salt Form.

Salt Form (S): Fraction of administered salt or ester form of the drug which is the active moiety.

Sensitivity Analysis: The practice of examining the relationship between a change in either clearance or volume of distribution and the corresponding change in the calculated plasma concentration.

SrCr: Serum Creatinine Concentration.

Steady State: Steady state is achieved when the rate of drug administration is equal to the rate of drug elimination.

t½: See Half-Life.

$t_{90\%}$: Time required to achieve 90% of steady state for phenytoin on a fixed dosing regimen in a patient with known values of Vd, Vm, and Km.

Tau (τ): See Dosing Interval.

$\tau - t_{in}$: Time from end of infusion to trough concentration when using a short infusion model.

TBW: See Total Body Weight.

T_d: Time of Dialysis.

T_{in}: Time required for drug to be infused or absorbed.

Tissue Concentration (C_t): Concentration of drug in the tissue.

Tissue Volume of Distribution (Vt): Apparent volume into which the drug appears to distribute following rapid equilibration with the initial volume of distribution.

Total Body Weight: Total weight of a patient usually used for obese patients.

Two-Compartment Model: Comprised of an initial, rapidly equilibrating volume of distribution (Vi) and an apparent second, more slowly equilibrating volume of distribution (Vt).

Unbound Vd: Volume of distribution based on the free or unbound plasma concentration.

Vd: See Volume of Distribution.

Vi: See Initial Volume of Distribution.

Vm: Maximum rate at which metabolism can occur.

Vt: See Tissue Volume of Distribution.

Volume of distribution (Vd): The apparent volume required to account for all the drug in the body if it were present throughout the body in the same concentration as in the sample obtained from the plasma.

90% t: Duration of therapy on a fixed dosing regimen which must be exceeded to assure that a measured phenytoin concentration represents steady state.

Appendix III:

SI Units and Symbols

Efforts to standardize the presentation of clinical laboratory data on an international level have resulted in the adoption of the Systeme International d'Unites (SI units). The uniform SI system will permit the interchangeability of information between nations and disciplines.

Name/Unit	Symbol
Meter	m
Kilogram	kg
Second	s
Mole	mol
Kelvin	K
Ampere	A
Candela	Cd
Square meter	m^2
Cubic meter	m^3
Newton (N)	$kg \cdot m \cdot s^{-2}$
Pascal (Pa)	$kg \cdot m^{-1} \cdot s^{-2}$ (N/m^2)
Joule (J)	$kg \cdot m2 \cdot s^{-2}$ ($N \cdot m$)
Kilogram per cubic meter	kg/m^3
Hertz (Hz)	s^{-1}

Osmolality Estimation (in mOsm/kg H_2O)

$$\text{Osmolality} = 2\left[Na^+ \text{ mEq/L}\right] + \frac{\left[\begin{array}{c}\text{glucose} \\ \text{(mg/dL)}\end{array}\right]}{20} + \frac{\left[\begin{array}{c}\text{BUN} \\ \text{(mg/dL)}\end{array}\right]}{3}$$

Blood Chemistry Reference Values

| Laboratory Test | Normal Reference Values | | Conversion Factor |
	Conventional Units	SI Units	
Acid phosphatase	0–5.5 U/L	0–90 nkat/L	16.67
ALT[a]	0–34 U/L	0–0.58 µkat/L[b]	0.01667
Albumin	4–6 gm/dL	40–60 gm/L	10
Alkaline phosphatase	30–120 U/L	0.5–2 µkat/L	0.01667
AST[c]	0–34 U/L	0.58 µkat/L	0.01667
Bilirubin			
Total	0.1–1 mg/dL	2–18 µmol/L	17.10
Direct	0–0.2 mg/dL	0–4 µmol/L	17.10
Blood urea nitrogen	8–18 mg/dL	3–6.5 mmol/L	0.3570
Calcium			
Total	9.2–11 mg/dL	2.3–2.7 mmol/L	0.2495
Unbound	4.0–4.8 mg/dL	1.0–1.2 mmol/L	0.2495
Carbon dioxide[d]	22–28 mEq/L	22–28 mmol/L	1
Chloride	95–105 mEq/L	95–105 mmol/L	1
Cholesterol			
LDL (low density lipoproteins)	50–190 mg/dL	1.30–4.90 mmol/L	0.02586
HDL (high density lipoproteins)	30–70 mg/dL	0.80–1.80 mmol/L	0.02586
Creatine kinase (CK)	0–130 U/L	0–2.16 µkat/L	0.01667
Creatinine	0.6–1.2 mg/dL	50–110 µmol/L	0.01667
Creatinine clearance	75–125 mL/min	1.24–2.08 mL/s	0.01667
GGT[e]	0–30 U/L	0–0.50 µkat/L	0.01667

(Continued)

	Normal Reference Values		
Laboratory Test	Conventional Units	SI Units	Conversion Factor
Globulin	2.3–3.5 gm/dL	23–35 gm/L	10
Glucose	70–110 mg/dL	3–6.1 mmol/L	0.055551
Iron			
Male	80–180 µg/dL	14–32 µmol/L	0.1791
Female	60–160 µg/dL	11–29 µmol/L	0.1791
Iron-binding capacity	250–460 µg/dL	45–82 µmol/L	0.1791
LH[f]	50–150 U/L	0.82–2.55 µkat/L	0.01667
Magnesium	1.6–2.4 mEq/L	0.80–1.20 mmol/L	0.500
Phosphate	2.5–5 mg/dL	0.80–1.60 mmol/L	0.3229
Potassium	3.5–5 mEq/L	3.5–5 mmol/L	1
Sodium	135–147 mEq/L	135–147 mmol/L	1
SGOT[g]	*See Aspartate aminotransferase (AST)*		
SGPT[h]	*See Alanine aminotransferase (ALT)*		
Triglycerides	<160 mg/dL	<1.80 mmol/L	0.01129
Uric acid	2–7 mg/dL	120–420 µmol/L	59.48

[a] ALT = Alanine aminotransferase.

[b] The unit katal (abbreviated kat) is a special name given to report catalytic activity. Thus, the new kat/L will replace international units per liter (U/L) as well as the various units of enzyme named after individuals (e.g., King-Armstrong units).

[c] AST = Aspartate aminotransferase.

[d] Bicarbonate plus CO_2.

[e] GGT = Gamma glutamyltransferase.

[f] LH = Lactate dehydrogenase.

[g] SGOT = Serum glutamate oxaloacetic transaminase.

[h] SGPT = Serum glutamate pyruvate transaminase.

Hematologic Laboratory Values

	Normal Reference Values		
Laboratory Test	Conventional Units	SI Units	Conversion Factor
ESR[a]			
Male	0–20 mm/hr	0–20 mm/hr	1
Female	0–30 mm/hr	0–30 mm/hr	1
Hemocrit			
Male	39%–49%	0.39–0.49 1[b]	0.01
Female	33%–43%	0.33–0.43 1	0.01
Hemoglobin			
Male	14–18 gm/dL	140–180 gm/L	10
Female	11.5–15.5 gm/dL	115–155 gm/L	10
MCH[c]	27–32 pg/RBC	27–32 pg	1
MCHC[d]	32–36 gm/dL	320–360 gm/L	10
MCV[e]	86–98 m^3/cell	86–98 fL[f]	1
Platelets	150,000–300,000/mm^3	1.5–3.0×10^{11}/L	.00001
RBC count[g]			
Male	4.3–5.9×10^6/mm^3	4.3–5.9×10^{12}/L	1
Female	3.5–5×10^6/mm^3	3.5–5×10^{12}/L	1
Reticulocyte count (adults)	0.1%–2.4%	0.001–0.024 1	0.001
WCB[h]	4500–11,000/mm^3	4.5–11×10^9/L	0.001

[a]ESR = Erythrocyte sedimentation rate.

[b]With the SI, the concept of number fraction replaces percentage. Thus for mass fraction, volume fraction, and relative quantities, the unit "1" is used to replace former units.

[c]MCH = Mean corpuscular hemoglobin.

[d]MCHC = Mean corpuscular hemoglobin concentration.

[e]MCV = Mean corpuscular volume.

[f]fL = Femtoliter; femto = 10^{-15}; pico = 10^{-12}; nano = 10^{-9}; micro = 10^{-6}; milli = 10^{-3}.

[g]RBC = Red blood cells; RBCs/Erythrocyte count.

[h]WBC = White blood cells; Leucocyte count.

Index